THE TAO OF HEALTH
THE WAY OF TOTAL WELL-BEING

Also by the author:

The Natural Healer's Acupressure Handbook
(Holt, Rinehart & Winston, Inc.;
   formerly entitled *The G-Jo Handbook*)

健
康
之
道

THE TAO OF HEALTH
THE WAY OF TOTAL WELL-BEING

MICHAEL BLATE
FOREWORD BY BARRY SULTANOFF, M.D.

FALKYNOR BOOKS

Davie, Florida 33314

    Grateful acknowledgment is made to Eastman Kodak Co.,
Inc., for permission to reproduce the author's photographs
found in Chapters 9 and 17.

Second edition/first impression

Library of Congress Cataloging in Publication Data

Blate, Michael   1938–

    The Tao of Health.

    Includes index.

    1. Health   2. Hygiene, Taoist. 3. Yin-yang

I. Title.

RA776.5.B55   613   78-50004

ISBN 0-916878-05-8

Photography—*Michael Blate*

Calligraphy—*Chow Chian-Chiu*

this book is for Gail . . .

*. . . and for Sri Sathya Sai Baba,
the Maker-of-Rainbows-to-Stand-Up-Straight.*

In motion, be as water;
at rest, like a mirror;
respond as an echo—
be subtle,
as though nonexistent

Taoistic aphorism

FOREWORD

At a time when the planet itself appears inevitably headed toward a healing crisis, *THE TAO OF HEALTH* offers a truly holistic way of viewing that progression and a clarification of how we may best attune ourselves to this process of evolution toward perfect health. Many have already become disillusioned with symptomatic health—the suppression of symptoms by any expedient means so to be spared, like the ostrich with his head in the sand, a painful confrontation with the reality of our progressive dis-ease. Instead, knowing that confrontation contains within it the seeds of positive change and realizing that each symptom that may emerge from the morass of our ignorance presents us with yet another opportunity for growth, we have chosen to meet the challenge of dis-ease with creative solutions. Health for us has come to mean much more than the absence (or *apparent* absence) of illness. It has become more and more synonymous with a process of awakening, an enlightenment. That we are now willing to face up to the painful work (or the "burning of karma," as the author puts it) required of us in this process of renewal raises a banner of optimism, a resounding *yes!,* heralding the New Age.

For there can be no doubt that the time of cleansing, of our individual "temples" as well as of our earthly Church/ Mother is upon us. It can be a most joyous time or a disaster. *THE TAO OF HEALTH* offers the reader some gentle guidance as he passes through this especially significant sector of his lifetime. Its practical philosophy, drawn from the ancient wisdom of the East, stands for the Westerner as a totem around which to rally through the challenges, struggles, and uncertainties which lie ahead. We begin to understand the wisdom of surrender, the strength in yielding, the "rightness" of following our intended path, our mission, our *dharma.* We come to more fully understand that health is a wholeness and a freedom that must be ours, and *will* be ours to the extent that we "go with" the natural forces that guide our lives. Each step along the way becomes its own reward: As we "give up" the foolish and inevitably fruitless task of overcoming, by means of our illusory ego, our self-generated obstacles, we paradoxically find the world "going our way."

Perhaps you've experienced moments (some call them "peak experiences") when your connectedness with your surroundings has been so perfect, when you've felt so "right" in your situation at that time and place, that *you could not even imagine* yourself in a more perfect or harmonious situation elsewhere. At such moments one tastes the sweet nectar of right *dharma.* Surrender is complete, the ego is quieted, the order and wisdom of the universe are understood. One stands humbly upon the path, feeling, if but for an instant, the peace of not-seeking and the gentle embrace of health and wholeness.

THE TAO OF HEALTH invites us to break off our love affair with the ego, to be wary of the karma that we may generate by carelessly overindulging its appetites. Understandably, we resist this offer. We enjoy the pleasures of a feast with friends, a night of lovemaking, a warm shoulder of praise or admiration. *I like my "attachments," dammit! I'm afraid to let go of them* . . . Yet there is within each of us the child who wishes to follow, not blindly or submissively, but joyously . . . *ahead, a path of daisies leads into the forest, and within that forest there is*—I sense this deeply—*nothing (no thing) to fear. Through the fog of my ignorance there is a beacon, a Light . . . I see it, sense it, but I need just a little nudge . . .*

That "little nudge" toward positive health, and ulti-
mately toward liberation through successive mini-enlightenments,
is what *THE TAO OF HEALTH* has to offer us. Its philosophy is a
clarification and a confirmation of what the inner "child" has
known all along: that there is no "getting away with" abuse to our
bodymind, for karma follows in our wake as an ever-present
witness, recording our thoughts, actions and behaviors, a mirror-
image of ourselves, reflecting our past whether we choose to
acknowledge it or not. Many of us have altered our course: We
have been "paying our dues" through better eating, more honest
relationships, meditation. We sense the immediacy of the changes
that are upon us, individually and collectively as part of the earth
community. We know that there is no "going against," only "going with." Respond we must, flexibly and wisely, if we are to survive and live our "full century."

May *THE TAO OF HEALTH* be for you an inspiration
as well as a pleasure. In its simplicity of presentation, may it lead
you, childlike, onward toward an honest, aware confrontation
with your karma, one that will free you more and more to follow
the path which is your *dharma*, your own path of service and enlightenment. And in its depth of message may it draw you ever
closer to an awakening and a way of life supportive to all lifeforms
and resonating with the universal consciousness.

May your path present you with all you will need to
grow. And may it be lined with daisies!

Barry Sultanoff, M.D.
Brockport, New York

ACKNOWLEDGMENTS

While many authors and teachers are to be thanked for the inspiration that culminated in *THE TAO OF HEALTH*, perhaps none is more important than the immortal Alan W. Watts. His writings and lectures have been, in my estimation, paramount in bringing the wisdom of the East to the studies, kitchens and bedrooms of the West.

In the preparation and publishing of this work, however, three names come immediately to mind:

Richard French—for his many hours of editing and for his invaluable advice in design and bookmaking;

Murray Spitzer—for his darkroom expertise and assistance;

Al Weisberg—for his part in the ink-on-paper process.

ABOUT THE PHOTOGRAPHS

Since, in the traditional Eastern point of view, all things are one thing—energy, manifested in countless, unique ways—I have approached illustrating *THE TAO OF HEALTH* with a sense of freedom and glee. Consequently, while some of the following photographs may be symbolic of passages in the text, this was incidental and not by design. My first consideration in their selection was pleasure—nothing more; these are some of my favorite works and I want to share them with you. Additional technical data may be found following the Afterword.

PROLOGUE

Before the beginning there was peace,
stillness, quiet, no-thing;
later—after time and names began—
this no-thing became Tao, the Way of All Things . . .

PART I

健康之道

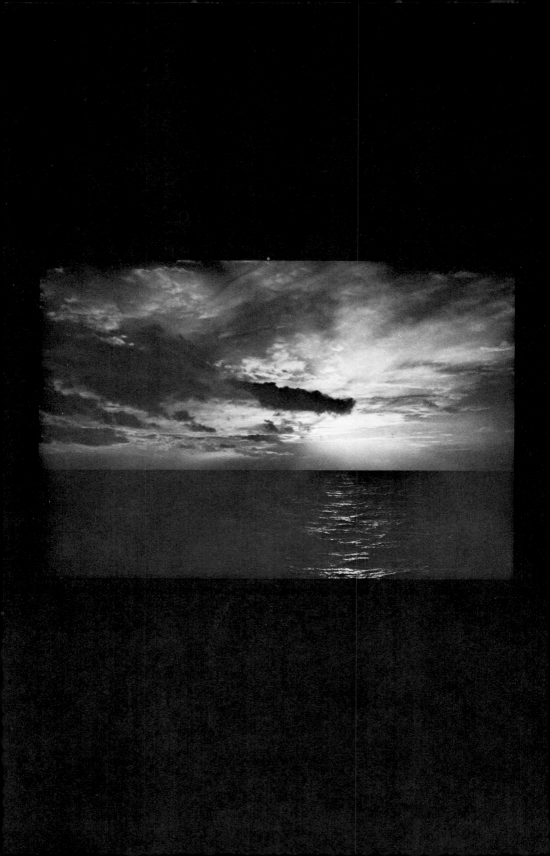

1

In the beginning, Tao wrenched itself in half;
light appeared—and heat, dryness, activity,
"heaven"—*the vacant sky and metaphysical realms . . .*
Yang! *Creation!*

Then darkness—
for how can light be noticed without darkness for contrast?
And cold—
for how can heat be otherwise measured?
And moisture, passivity, the planets and physical realm . . .
Yin! *Inseparable reaction to creation!*

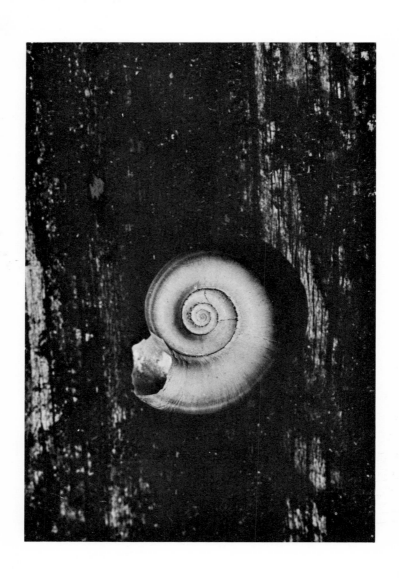

2

Tao—now with two identities instead of none—
became distressed in reaction to its division:
> *Whose personality shall reign supreme—*
> *that of yang or yin?*
> *Each is essential to the other*
> *as a reflection is to a mirror . . .*

Tao is exactly half yang and half yin—
never more, never less;
here, a picture of Tao's dilemma:

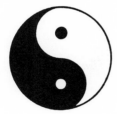

> *Tao—the universe, its forms and realms—*
> *is represented by the complete circle;*
> *yang, the light, tries "overwhelming" yin, the dark;*
> *yin occupies the space vacated by yang . . .*

Each is indomitable—
yet each exercises some control over the other—
represented by the small "eye" in either half—
but thereby allows the other the same influence,
the same partial control, upon itself:
Half is but half, wherever residing, however divided.

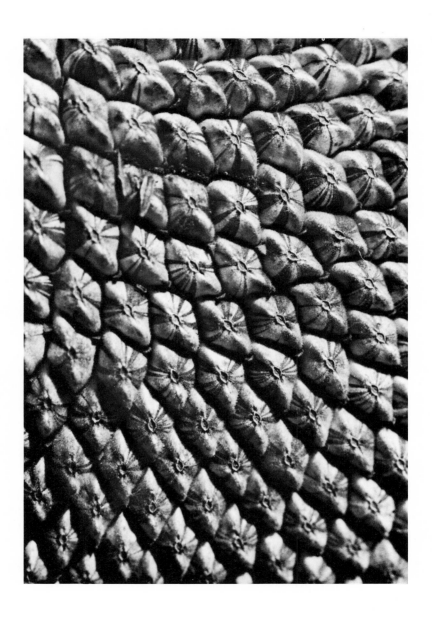

3

Within the circle of Tao, an action—
such as "pushing inward" at one place—
must create a reaction of "pulling out" in another:
For every action, an identical reaction must someplace occur.

The "conflict" for dominance between yang and yin—
a constant activity, unceasing in nature—
generates *energy* as the necessary reaction
from the friction upon each interface
where yang and yin meet;
yet where yang and yin meet—no chaos:
When the ocean pushes forward on one shore,
it ebbs away from another . . .

Each thing in the universe—*everything—*
visible, invisible, tangible, ethereal—
is produced from this *"force with a thousand names,"*
this vital essence, this **bioenergy.**

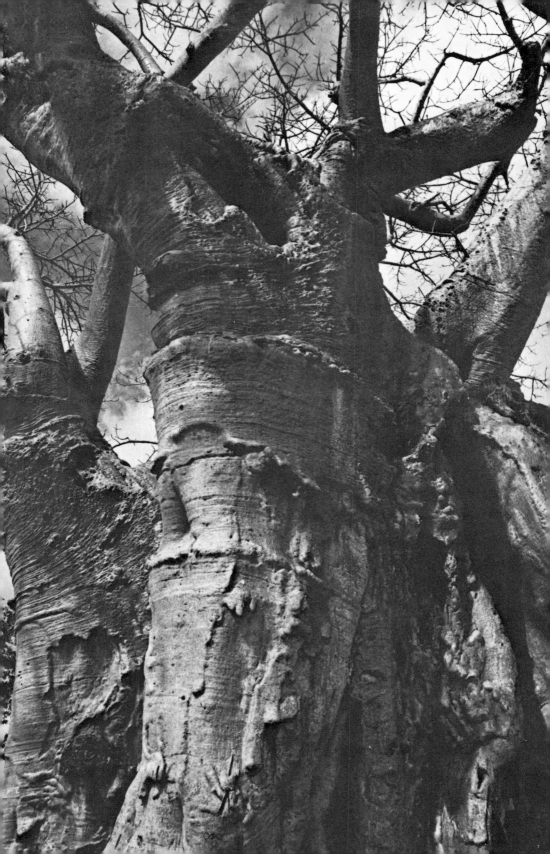

4

Tao is constant, as are yang and yin—
bioenergy, too, cannot be destroyed,
but "vibrates" between yang and yin
in methodical cycles—
while the tiny acorn and the towering oak
are unalike, yet essential for each other's creation,
so each *cycle of change* may be "divided"
into **five separate—though crucial—steps or phases:**

       Birth *of the cycle;*
       surging upward—*rapid growth, "childhood";*
       peaking—*maturity or "adulthood";*
       falling downward—*decay, "old age";*
       death, *and the next cycle's rebirth.*

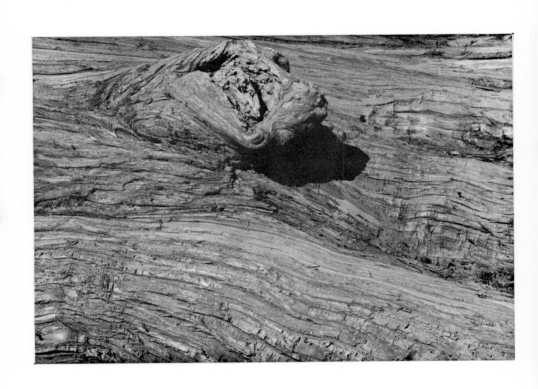

5

Between yang and yin is found bioenergy—
the force from which all things are manifested;
thus, no thing is purely yang, the light,
nor anything totally yin, the dark.

The tension and friction between yang and yin
trying to unite without loss of personal identity,
this is the "sexual activity" that generates bioenergy;
and bioenergy—*during its first, five-step cycle of change*—
created the **five elements of the universe:**
>In its *birth phase* arose **wood**—*all growing matter;*
>in its *surging upward phase,* **fire**—*air, gases* . . .
>in its *mature adult phase,* **earth**—*dirt, soil* . . .
>in its *decay phase,* **metal**—*all inorganic matter;*
>in the *death/rebirth phase,* **water**—*all moisture.*

Each thing, each activity, found in the universe
is a unique formula of elements interacting;
thus, yang and yin are everythings' parents
and each form or activity is related to all others.

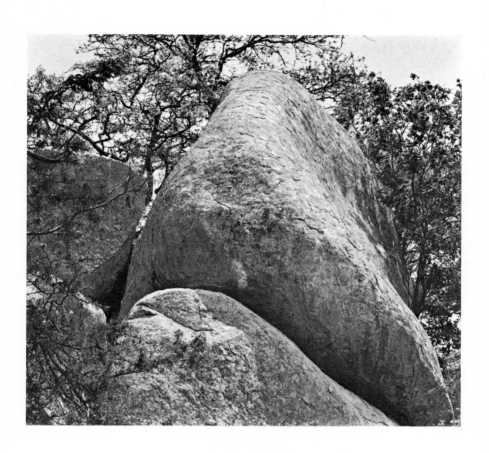

6

A misty cloud seems unlike a rock,
the fire seems unlike a tree:
Each element of the universe has a vast range of vibration—
the more "slowly" a combination of elements vibrates,
the more **"condensed"** its form becomes
and the more *like yin* it is said to be;
the more "rapidly" an elemental combination vibrates,
the more *like yang*—the more **"free"**—it is said to be.

The rock: *more yin than the cloud*—
the fire: *more yang than the tree;*
yang and *yin* are words of comparison,
ways of describing which of any two things—
which of any two activities—
is more free or condensed than the other.

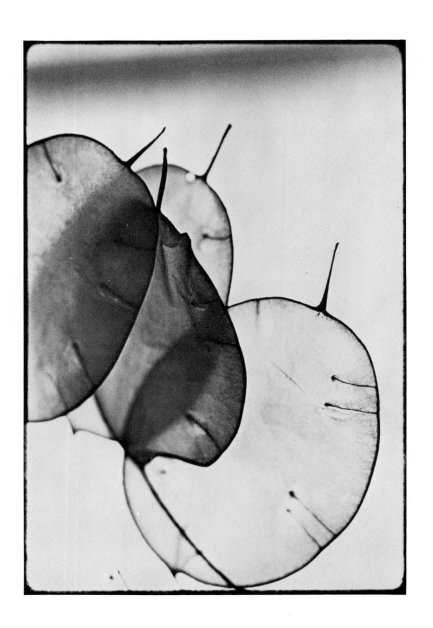

7

Within the universe—*no voids!* Only bioenergy—
some visibly condensed, the rest more subtle and free—
each form is an eye in yang, the light,
each form is an island in the "sea of free bioenergy"—
the space between atoms is filled with yang energy,
the eagle is immersed in the sky . . .

Yang gives "life" to condensed bioenergy,
yin provides the vessel for yang;
the hardest metal is touched by the fire of activity,
no thought exists without a degree of form.

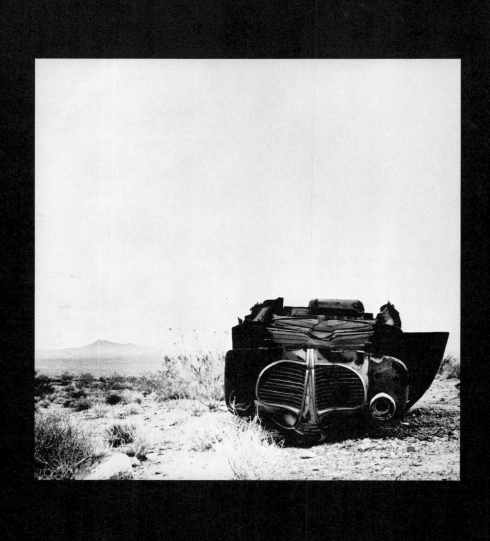

8

Yang and yin,
bioenergy, its five elemental arrangements
and all their constantly changing forms—
each, an unnatural disturbance in Tao;
every physical form yearns for freedom,
each seeks its own return path to no-thingness;
evolution—*the return path to peace*—is ceaseless:
Yin surrenders form to yang, reversing creation—
the rock decays, the mountain is liberated into dust . . .

Beyond bioenergy, beyond yang and yin,
the nature of Tao is harmonious peace—
Tao wrenching itself into halves changed nothing:
The circle contains perfection and unity—
division only rearranged Tao, creating an illusion,
the ***maya***—*the deception*—from which all forms are built,
the bottomless well from which all actions are drawn.

Yet until Tao accepts the inevitable
and surrenders *both* identities, yang and yin,
nothing is ever lost in the universe—only rearranged—
for where could it possibly go?

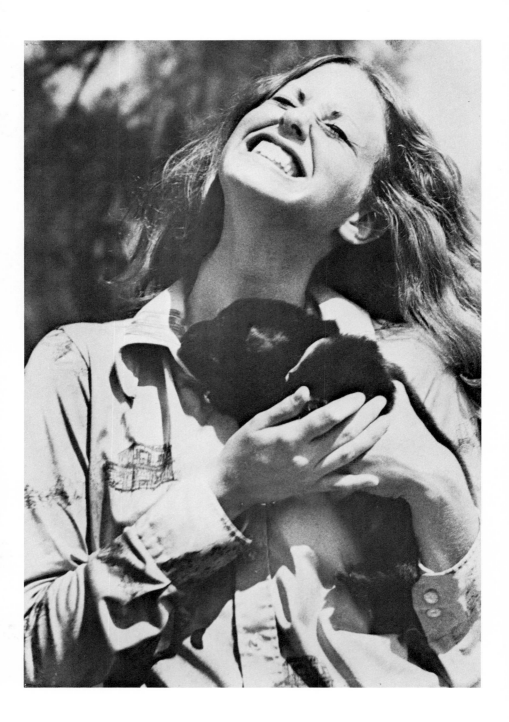

9

I am a human being;
I am a relatively yin manifestation
immersed and submerged in relative yang;
I am less condensed—less yin—than the rock
upon which I may sit and rest—
I am more vital, more alive, more yang than brother rock,
further evolved, further liberated, more free . . .

But I am less alive than the ocean of yang bioenergy
that pervades me, interfusing me to my environment;
from this sea of energy I attract the vitality
to continue, for the moment, as my uniquely condensed form.

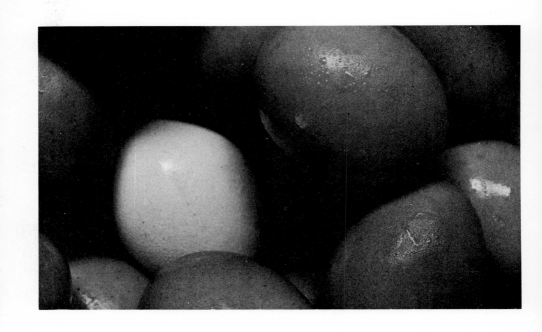

10

I am one point of view of reality;
my viewpoint—if added to all others in the universe,
animal, vegetable, human, inorganic, metaphysical—
reveals Tao, the Perfect, the Circle, the Whole . . .

There is only perfection and oneness,
yet I cannot sense the fullness of Tao
just as no cell of mine totally senses the being with my name:
Each cell is a **microcosm**—*a tiny model or pattern*—
of its **macrocosm**—*the being it helps to shape.*

Energy form upon energy form upon energy form,
cycle within cycle within cycle—
I am a microcosm of Tao's creation of the universe,
ceaselessly duplicating within me the five steps of change.

I cannot stand alone, separate from my surroundings—
I am totally subject to the order of the universe,
totally ruled by the natural laws governing my environment;
I can surrender to these laws and live healthfully—
in complete harmony—for a full century;
or I can live in ignorance—often *ignore*-ance—of,
even in flagrant rebellion against, my natural confines
and suffer to the extent of my violation.

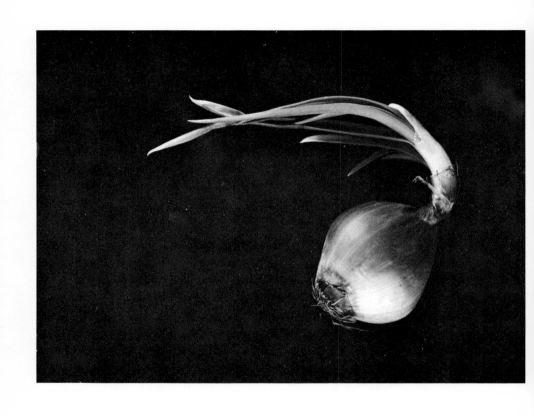

11

I am an egg-shaped mass of condensed bioenergy;
within this *auric ovoid,* this **aura** of bioenergy,
are the various "parts" of my being,
arranged—like a rainbow—in layers or **sheaths**.

The "yolk" of this auric egg—
the most condensed and deeply buried part of my aura—
is my **vital organs**—
liver, lungs, spleen-pancreas, heart and kidneys—
surrounded and protected by the rest of my organs and *body.*

Enclosing and permeating the physical body is my **mind**—
my rational and psychoemotional sheath;
more subtle, still—most yang and free—is my **soul**:
A pinpoint of purest "consciousness"—
expanded, my soul permeates my **bodymind**
the way a flame pervades a matchstick,
fusing all these sheaths into the vital being that I am.

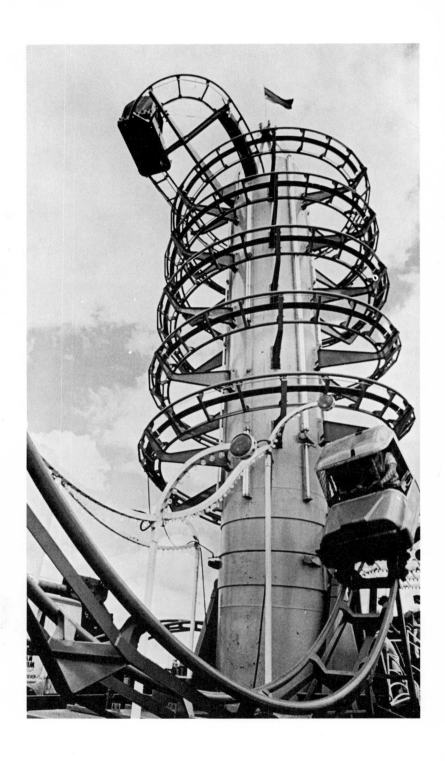

12

My yin-like presence in the sea of yang
attracts free bioenergy for my continued vitality
the way standing in sunlight attracts my shadow;
my soul—most yang of my auric sheaths—
is connected to each of my organs
by a vast network of *energy viaducts*—
my pathway of **meridians:**
Free bioenergy flows, like a river of life,
along these meridians—touching each organ in sequence—
moved by the tension between my own yang and yin.

As wind meeting leaves makes them dance in excitement,
so free bioenergy animates each of my organs—
reaching my heart, bioenergy makes it beat with vitality . . .

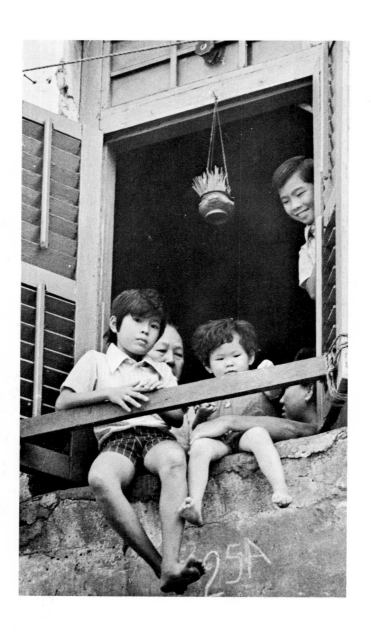

13

Between conception and birth,
the activities of each budding and blossoming organ
created the rest of my bodymind in response to their frolic:
  Bones sprouted in response to my kidneys' activities;
  muscles and tendons, from the action of my liver;
  blood and its circulatory system—from my heart;
  flesh—that which fills otherwise unoccupied body space—
  arose in reaction to my spleen-pancreas;
  skin, from my lungs;
  brainstem, nervous system and **chakras**—
  centers and reservoirs of my psychic energy—
  from the activities along my spinal meridian.

Each bodily part is related to its "home organ"
the way a child is permanently related to its parents.

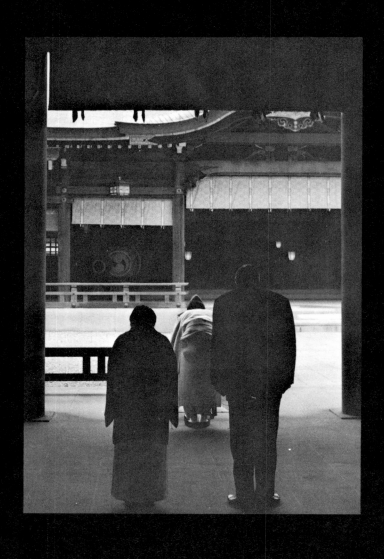

14

Just as a child cannot be conceived
without the activities of two parents,
so the five vital organs have their own, natural mates:
  The kidneys are paired with the *urinary bladder*;
  the liver with the *gall bladder*;
  the heart with the *small intestine*;
  the spleen-pancreas with the *stomach*;
  the lungs with the *large intestine*;
  and the spinal meridian with the *frontal meridian*.

And just as the activities of a husband or wife
must subsequently affect those of the partner,
so each organ's actions have a direct bearing
on the quality and functions of its mate.

The interaction of these pairs of organs—
their harmonies, antipathies and disagreements—
creates the constantly changing "opinions"
that influence the flow of my free bioenergy.

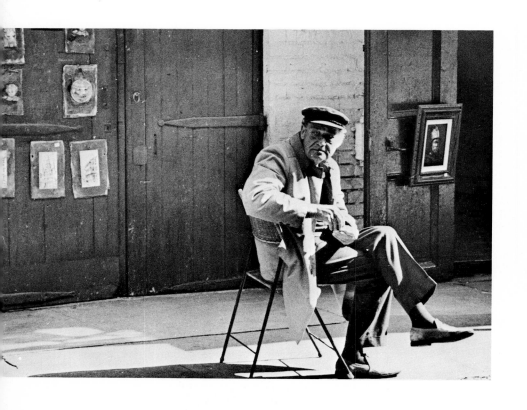

15

Bioflow courses along my meridians
then returns to my soul after vitalizing each organ,
completing its circuit, sustaining my life;
but I am in a constant state of activity—
thinking, digesting, sensing, doing—
and each activity, as its necessary reaction,
depletes some of my bioflow on its way back to my soul,
driving it out through my aura's "boundries,"
into the ocean of energy from which it was drawn.

As my free bioenergy becomes depleted I sense **hunger**—
the yearning to have my bioflow replenished,
to have it restored to its own unique standard:
> Depletion of my heart and lungs causes *smothering*,
> creating within me the hunger for air;
> activities depleting my kidneys cause *thirst*,
> while depletion of my liver and spleen-pancreas
> stimulates a hunger for *"solid food"*;
> mental activities create **boredom**—
> the hunger *to relax, to become mentally tranquil.*

Each "food"—solid, liquid, air, "entertainment"—
liberates free bioenergy at a "speed" and "intensity"
most compatible with the organs each feeds.

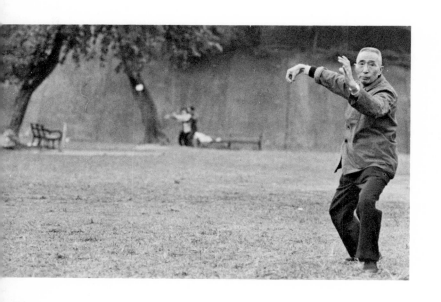

16

Each food, each energy source, that I digest
has an increasing or decreasing effect—
a yang or yin effect—
on the beat and the balance of my bioflow.

The more perfectly my bioflow is balanced
between excess and deficiency, between yang and yin,
the less free bioenergy I need to extract from my food
to maintain the harmony and stability
of my own, unique pulse.

But until each hunger is satisfied (or somehow controlled—
free will, meditation, special training or techniques . . .)
I cannot continue in a good state of health:
Each organ's hunger creates a **"warp"** in reaction—
a tension causing that organ to malfunction—
which then affects the rest of my bodymind.

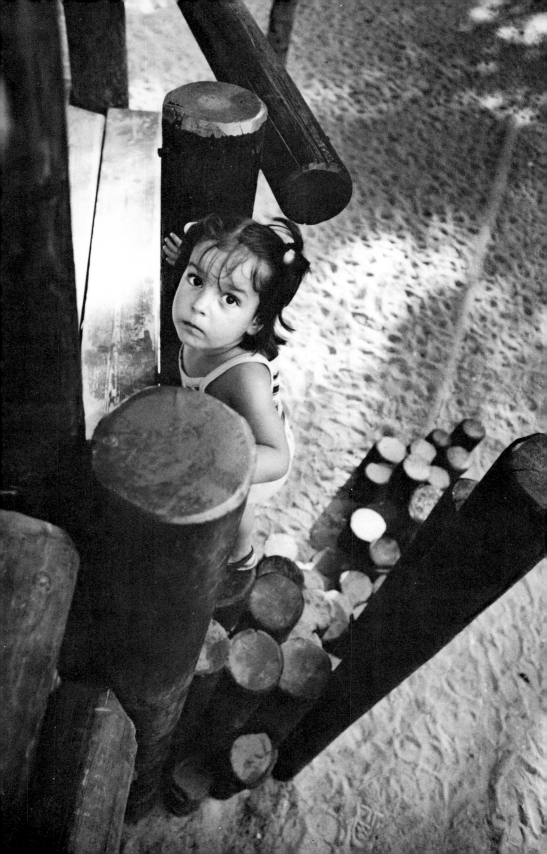

17

At birth, I was totally helpless;
open and yielding to all that surrounded me
I was unable to distinguish the difference
between the outer and my own, inner environment;
I held no values nor judgments—
animal comforts were my guides.

Then: *a hunger not instantly satisfied—anger! Fear . . .*
A pleasure denied me too long—sorrow . . . grief . . .
Yet I stubbornly clung to what I sensed was my due—
remembering, learning . . .thinking and judging . . .

As rowing a boat across a still pond
generates whirlpools in the wake of the oars,
so each cycle of change—more a yang phenomenon—
meeting my resistance and hesitancy—more yin—
created an *experience* from the friction of meeting.

Each experience—each whirlpool of my reaction to change—
developed, then nurtured, the idea and notion
that something was *me* and the rest of it *not-me*;
now angry, now fearful, now threatened and tiny,
thus it was that my **ego**—*my sense of self*—was born.

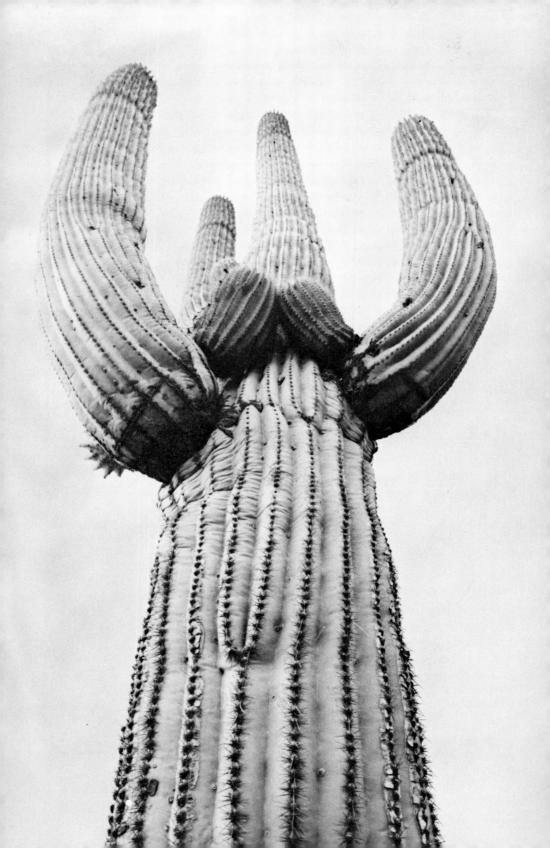

18

My ego—a protective response—arose as a buffer
from the barrage of changing conditions,
a device to shelter and surround me,
to help keep me from duplicating painful experiences.

My animal feelings of infancy days
were finally suppressed into judgments and opinions,
then began manifesting as my **personality**—
personality is like a balloon;
ego, like the heat that inflates it.

Yet the experiences forming my ego and personality—
like whirlpools which cannot constantly spin,
but seek to be filled as their natural course—
must either be totally released from my memory
or lodge themselves someplace in my bodymind
as *unreacted reactions pending completion of their cycles.*

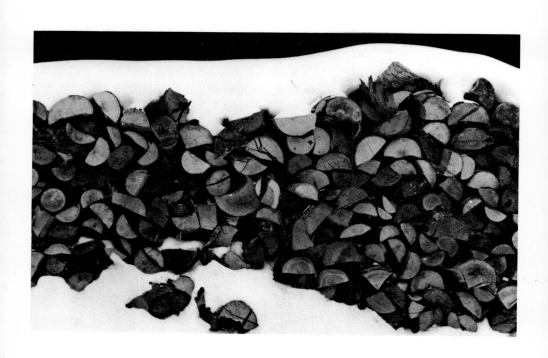

19

Ego—the main "component" of mind—
belongs to the body as a fragrance belongs to a fish;
though my bodymind is a whole, I have separate organs,
and, as a hoarder conceals his riches in caches,
I stash my incomplete reactions to change
deeply—as tensions and warps—in my various organs:
> My kidneys receive unfinished *fear and sexual orgasm*;
> my liver, the remains of *depression and anger*;
> my heart stores unreacted *joy and sorrow*;
> my lungs—*anguish and resentment* I've had to repress;
> my spleen-pancreas is the trove and receptacle
> for *stubborness and empathy* I have yet to express.

That which I have stashed as warps in my organs
provides motivation for all that I seek—
these stashes are the bases of my *emotional drives*:
> Kidneys release *caution and prudence*;
> liver, *aggressiveness and "pushing-forwardness"*;
> heart—*exuberance and "love of living"*;
> lungs release *concern and solicitude*;
> spleen-pancreas—*sympathy and persistence.*

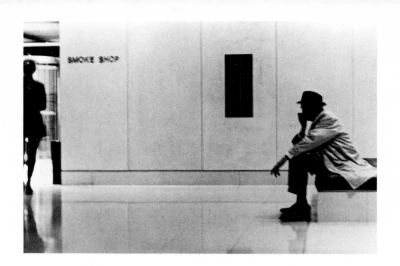

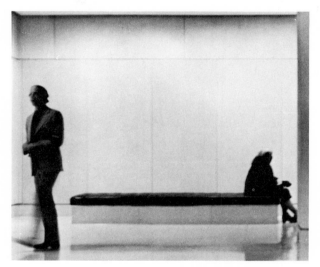

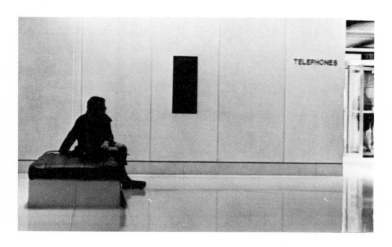

20

At its most healthy, at its most useful,
my ego is a balanced combination of thrusts and restraints,
an orchestration of emotional drives in activity;
but a surge or depletion of bioflow to an organ—
whatever the reason, whatever the source—
causes an *emotional outburst* to occur in reaction

My outburst may be suppressed and stashed in its organ—
causing further "internal" pressure and distress—
or be poured forth and vented, relieving the imbalance;
yet an outburst or "inburst" must always arise
as an emotional drive becomes thwarted in its expression.

From my basic drives gone berserk,
as my ego is thwarted, as my ego is threatened,
from this, all emotional "feelings" arise—
my angers, my fears . . . my grieving and sorrows—
as each organ pours forth its pent-up stashes . . .

The more tumultuous my emotional reactions,
the more powerfully they affect the balance of my bioflow
and the state of my organ/meridian system.

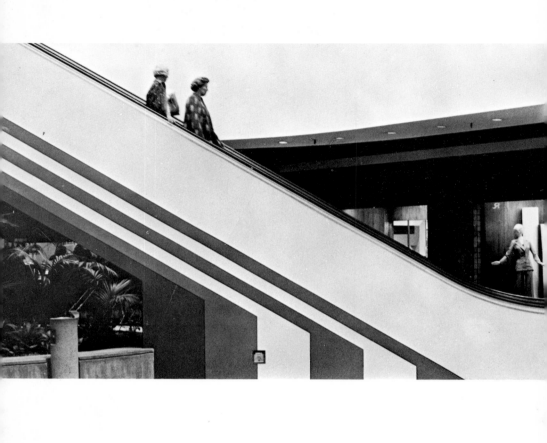

21

In the universe there are no coincidences—
every action arises from a previous action,
every action is truly a *re*action:
Yang and yin are Tao's reaction—
had Tao not divided, no yang nor yin,
nor bioenergy nor world of illusion . . .

At any moment I am where I am—
not by coincidence—but by my own reactions,
from feelings and yearnings and fears in my past,
from logical choices that I "had to make";
I am where I am because of my **karma**—
my self-generated accumulated destiny—
the path along which my stashed reactions
have lured me, have coaxed me,
have goaded or driven me . . .

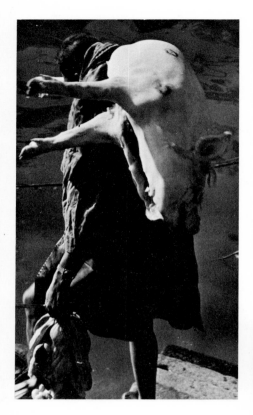

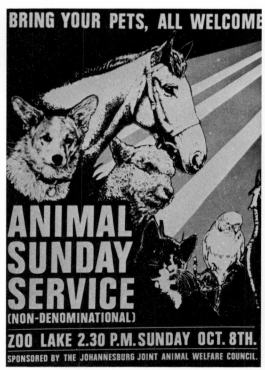

22

In the universe, neither good nor bad exist,
neither right nor wrong, nor just and unjust—
only yang and yin and their natural laws;
yet karma—
generated by activities contrary to the laws of nature—
seems "good" or "bad."

But depending upon my intentions—*and self-judgments*—
the same activity may hold different karmic repercussions:
       I may kill a creature by accident,
         and that was *its* karma—I was merely an instrument;
         or I may kill that creature because it is suffering;
         or because I hunger for its flesh;
         or because it attacks me;
         or even because I yearn to kill . . . something.

By acting deliberately against the natural laws
I generate more karma than by acting in ignorance—
thus, in self-protection, I avoid seeking knowledge—
or ignore what I sense—until its time is correct,
for ignorance, once revealed, becomes highly karmic
if an activity is repeated after I understand its consequence;
and the karma I generate from an unwise activity
is gentled to the extent of its selfless intentions.

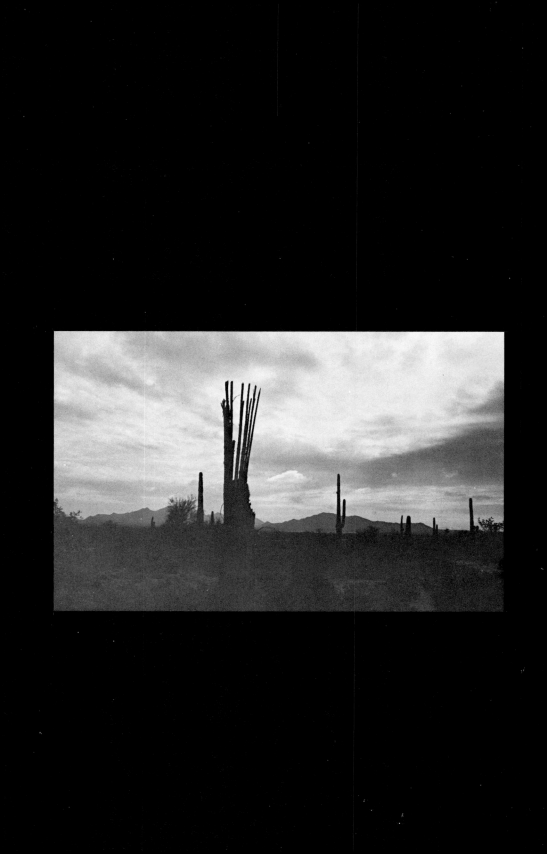

23

As sand blowing across the desert is without consequence,
so activity without interpretation—and without memory—
is likewise without karma;
yet I remember nearly all my activities—
consciously or not—
and interpret them, based on the values my ego has built,
finding some to be wanting or "sinful" or "wrong,"
while others are judged as unquestionably "right!"

Though I may share a karmic experience with another,
his karma is his—not mine, not ours—and my karma is mine;
I—my own karmic jury and executioner—
determine the impact of each thought and deed,
then generate *guilt* for the wrong ones and *pride* for the right.

Pride and guilt: These are the yang and yin faces
of my emotions—stashed or reacted—
whose consequences, when buried in my various organs,
becomes my karma, the force
that propels me to their completion or *"burning."*

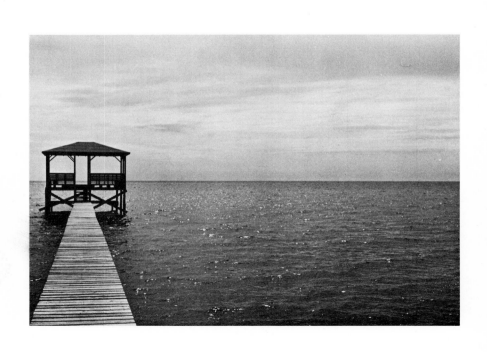

24

My bodymind is constantly, subtly, changing,
reflecting the weight of my karmic burden,
mirroring the imbalance of my organ/meridian system;
yet my soul remains both free and unmuddied,
protected from contamination by the "filtering" action
of the *karmic-intuitive* sheath of my aura.

As personality—the manifestation—is to my ego,
so *intuition*, and **conscience**—*the voice of my soul*—
are the manifestation of karma, the force.

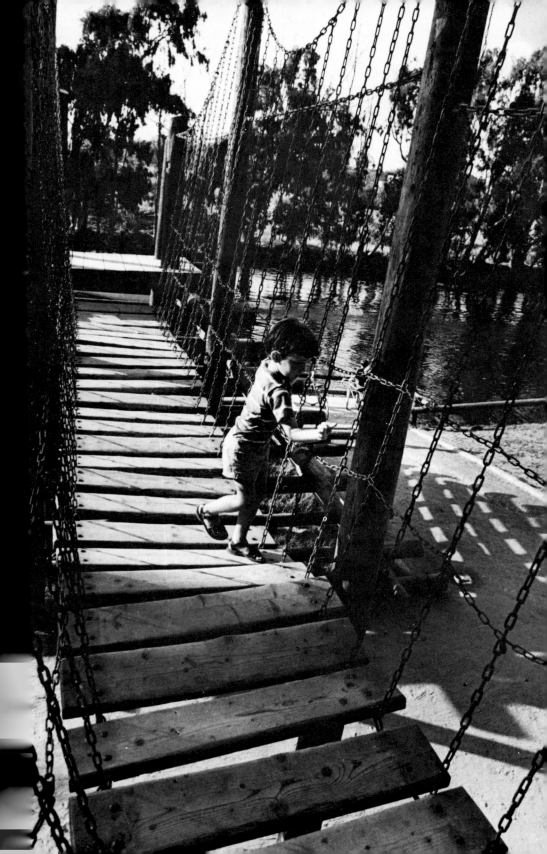

25

Ego, a response to fear, arose to insure my survival—
stripped, as an onion may be stripped of its layers,
*ego holds but a single seed—**fear of death**.*

From this single fear, all other fears—and quests—arise.

Death—a relative, step-by-step phenomenon;
its most dramatic phase, physical death,
occurs when my bioflow can no longer complete its circuit
between the yang of my soul and the yin of my organs.

The interplay between my yang and yin
binds my cells to each other,
fuses my soul to my bodymind,
welds each auric sheath into a single unit;
dying, this adhesion first falters, then loosens—
I hyper-relax; my organ/meridian system quickly unwarps,
*draining away **most—but not all**—of my karma,*
easing the tension, the binding, between my auric sheaths . . .

As a drop of rain must return to the earth,
so, upon dying, the principal part of my free bioenergy
returns through my aura to the vast sea of yang.

26

Nothing is lost within the realms of the universe:
As a sleeper awakens, so, at the moment of physical death,
I—a subtler, yet more yang, more alive, consciousness—
step out of one realm, step *into* another;
bioenergy, while constantly changing, cannot be destroyed—
I cannot become simply nothing
when only moments earlier I was something . . .

My physical life is a brief punctuation
in an eternal continuum of countless dimensions:
Just as mind can exist in the same space as body,
and as soul can permeate the space of the bodymind,
so my karma remaining from the life I just quit—
my "leftover" ego, my still-unfinished reactions—
occupies space that is already occupied in the vast sea of yang,
an auric archetype, a pattern, a karmic "cocoon"
around which will be manifested my next *incarnation.*

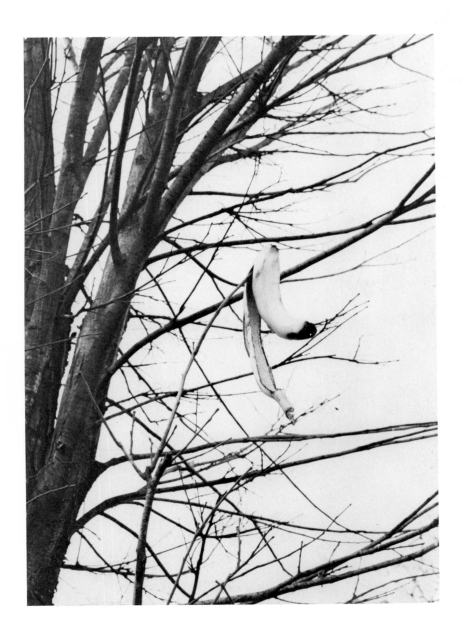

27

I reincarnate countless times yet have but a single life—
one existence, many egos, many personalities,
many opportunities to burn—and regenerate—karma.

The apple tree sleeps through many winters
but blossoms forth each springtime—
each incarnation is a harvest of karmic "fruit,"
each is dropped as it ripens;
yet the "tree"—my soul—
remains the source of each incarnation, each bodymind,
surviving harvest after harvest and life after life . . .

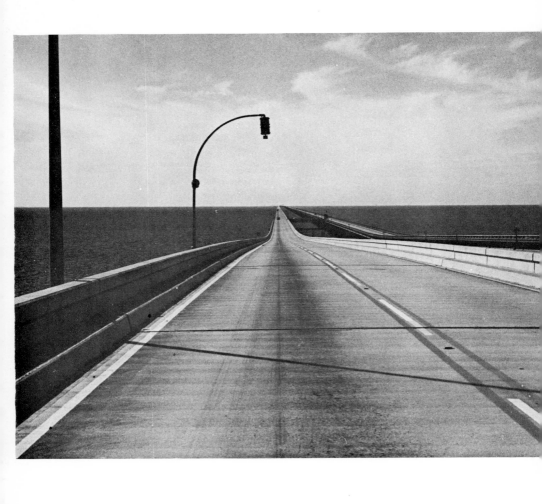

28

Bored and restless, I wander in another realm,
unfinished, earthly "business" nagging at me until . . .
. . . I reincarnate into the perfect time, the perfect place,
the perfect situation in the perfect body,
for the opportunity to burn my most pressing karma—
into familiar circumstances and settings,
among old friends and old enemies,
old teachers and followers,
old parents and children . . .

The more pressing my karma—
the more emotionally attached I have remained to this realm—
the faster the next "me" is manifested.

Karma shapes my ego and personality
to fit and conform to my surroundings—
I am a perfect reflection of my karmic burden;
yet I cannot *see* my karma because I *am* my karma;
I may believe myself to have unlimited choice,
yet just as a fish in a small bowl can choose freely
that part of his container he wishes to occupy,
he is totally confined to his vessel as I am to my karma.

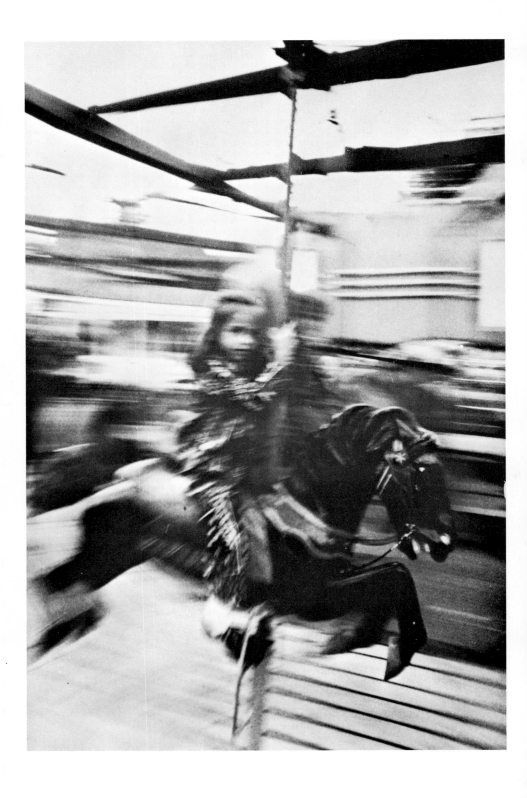

29

Waking from each night's sleep, my dreams—
while serving a useful purpose of releasing emotional tension—
are quickly forgotten as daylight returns;
so it is with reincarnation and karma:
I begin each bodymind free in memory, free of "facts,"
free from conscious guilt and pride,
free to wander my same path again . . .

Yet as surely as a bubble—
trapped beneath the surface of a pond—
must either rise or remain in a state of distress,
so I evolve toward a single goal:
to break the karmic cycle of birth, death and rebirth—
to free myself from the miseries of aging,
the monotony of relearning old lessons,
the trauma of birth and the terror of dying . . .

Freedom from this is the goal of my life.

PART II

健康之道

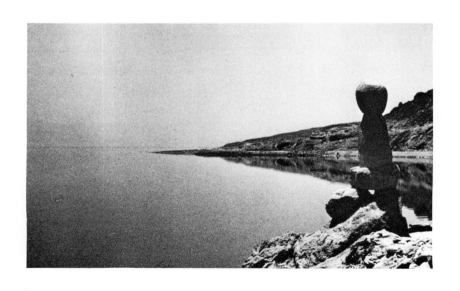

30

The bright moon, no clouds, a calm lake—
there! A perfect reflection . . .

Good health—the reflection of harmony
existing between soul, mind and body—
occurs when I live peacefully within my environment,
when my bioflow is balanced between yang and yin.

But as an image cast upon a still lake
may easily be shattered—
a breeze, the falling rain, a leaping fish—
so the delicate balance of my bioflow
may be disturbed by **eight, basic abuses:**
>**improper or excessive foods and beverages;**
>**imbalanced sexual activity;**
>**psychoemotional extremes**—*anger, joy, grief . . .*
>**external extremes**—*injuries, stings, bites . . .*
>**meteorological extremes**—*rain, wind, cold,*
>>*pollution, astrological dischord . . .*
>
>**internal parasites;**
>**poisoning by extreme yang or yin**—*drugs, herbs . . .*
>**"plagues" and epidemics**—*germs or viruses.*

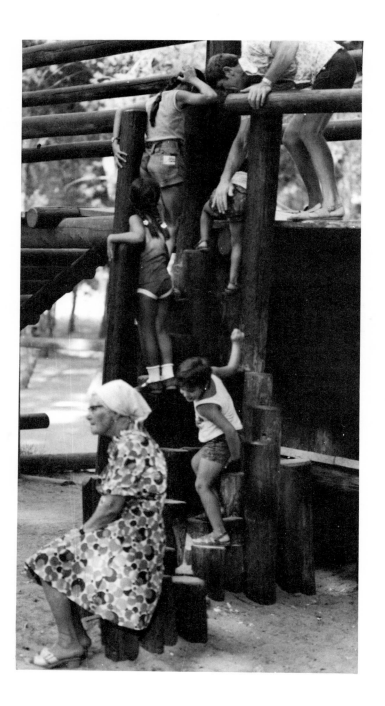

31

There exists—beyond the basic, eight abuses—
a **ninth "abuse,"** without which poor health cannot occur:
karmic readiness—the accumulated results of my failure
to completely respond to, and flow with, and adjust to,
constantly changing situations and surroundings.

I may appear to respond easily to abuses,
moving through them, and beyond,
as if they were non-existent;
yet each abuse adds its burden
to the existing state of my organs' warp,
causing my bioflow to react—*surging, lulling*—
until my ability to respond bcomes impaired.

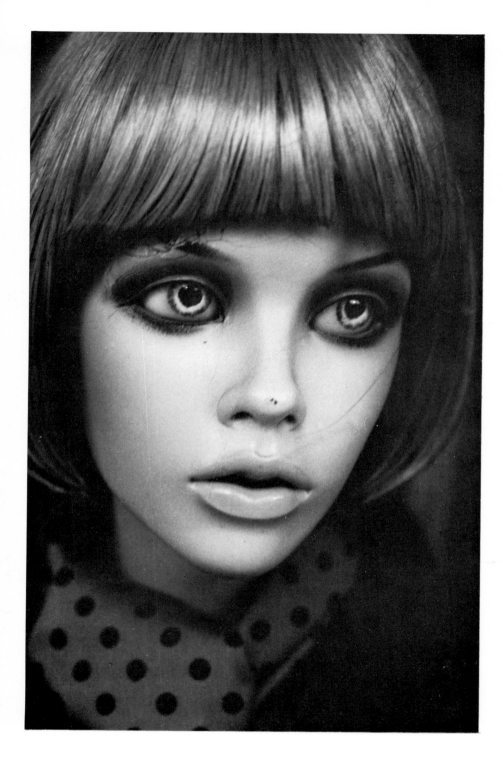

32

Just as a reaction must always follow an action,
so, when my bioflow surges above—or falls below—
its ideal "operational level,"
a *symptom* of illness must manifest itself—
however subtly or overtly—
someplace in my bodymind.

Yet while there are countless symptoms of poor health,
there exists but one illness, alone:
imbalanced bioflow throughout my organ/meridian system.

All bioenergy seeks freedom and ease;
the more condensed the bioenergy form,
the more *dis*-eased it is—
my bodymind—relatively condensed bioenergy—
is in a constant state of dis-ease.

The bodymind in the physical realm:
An imperfect vehicle in an imperfect state,
suffering many symptoms of the single dis-ease . . .

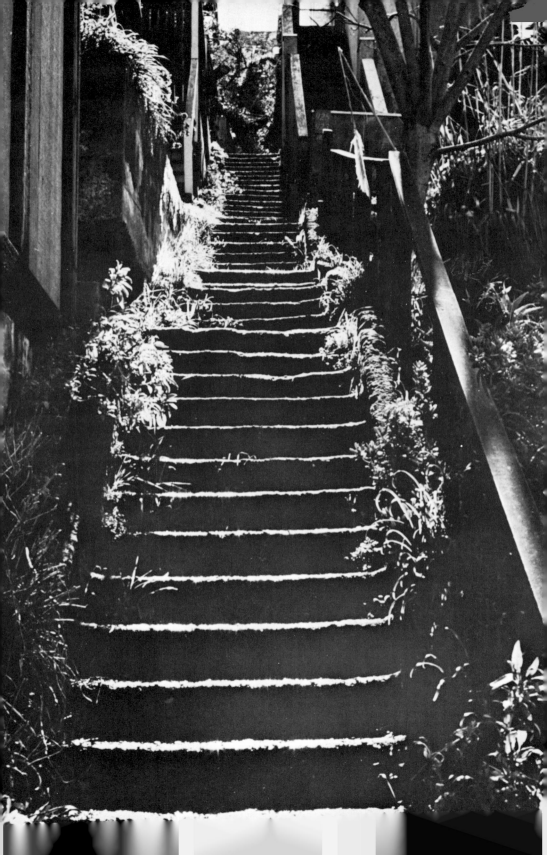

33

The path of dis-ease follows a logical course:
      First, abuse—
      my bioflow surges or lulls in reaction;
      then **"acupoints"**—*tiny defense "mechanisms"*
      found, by the hundreds, along my meridians—
      counter-react by "clenching" or "slackening,"
      trying to restore and maintain
      the delicate balance of my bioflow;
      as abuse continues, the acupoints are "over-ridden,"
      and imbalance floods my organ/meridian network;
      as imbalanced bioflow reaches an organ,
      that organ reacts by warping or kinking—
      the karma, now stashed, awaits its burning.

Just as a vessel can overflow
only after it has been filled beyond its capacity,
so my dis-ease precedes its **symptom syndrome**—
the related group of signals that dis-ease has manifested itself;
the specific organ—and the way it is warped—
determine the area of my bodymind
where the symptom syndrome will manifest most grossly.

The process may take moments or months—
the variables are *time* and *intensity*—
but the path of dis-ease remains the same.

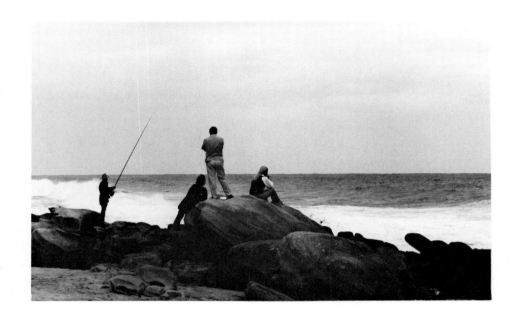

34

The interplay of environmental forces—outer and inner—
upon my organ/meridian system,
produces the conflicts that affect and afflict
the harmony and balance of my bioflow;
the condition of bioflow coursing along its pathway
influences—no, *controls*—
my every activity, my every perception;
my state of awareness, my "level" of consciousness—
the "reality" I perceive through my senses—
is totally dependent upon the state of my bioflow.

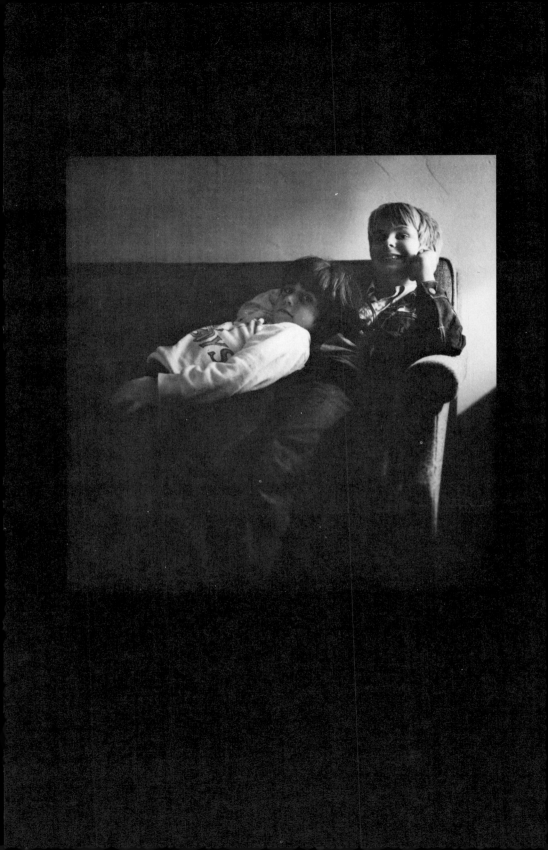

35

Each bodily part (*eyes, teeth, nails, hair, tongue . . .*)
grew outward—a "child"—
from the activities of one pair of organs or another;
if a child is injured, or somehow afflicted,
its "parents"—the home organs—must also suffer;
but if one—or a pair of—home organs is warped,
a child or children will not necessarily—
though easily *might*—
manifest symptoms of the parental distress.

A symptom syndrome—"physical" or "mental"—
may manifest itself in sites
far removed from its home pair of organs;
yet just as each bodily part has its parents,
so each symptom syndrome has an organ for home.

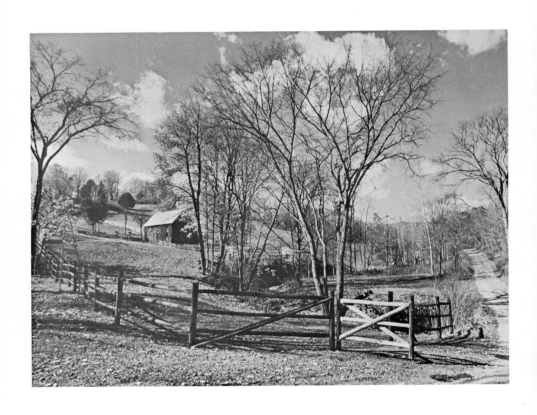

36

Each of my organs has its precarious season,
its time in the annual cycle of change
when that organ is most sensitive, most active—
its time of tenderness and vulnerability;
the karma from incompleted reactions to change
is most easily released, most easily burned,
during that organ's weakest time of the year.

Just as each organ has its sensitive part of the year,
so, too, each has its special time of the day—
those hours when that organ's characteristics—
vibrant, chaotic, sluggish—
are most visibly reflected throughout my bodymind;
thus, I feel better—or worse—
during or two hours of the day,
and in one or another part of the year.

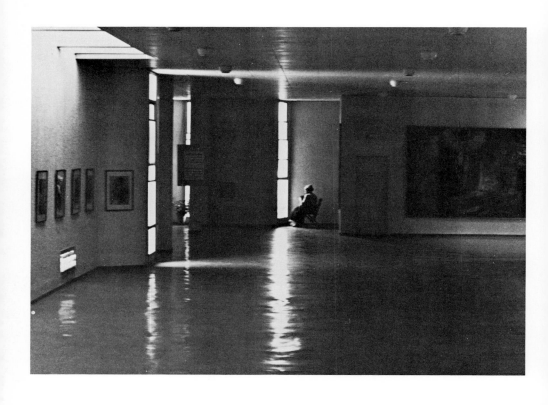

37

The roots of each symptom syndrome—
including "accidental" injuries—
are found in the *karmic/intuitive sheath* of my aura;
in good health, I can respond freely to all manner of change,
surrender peacefully to even harsh abuse,
without seriously disrupting my balance of bioflow.

Yet I have at least one pair of **"target organs"**—
those permanently weakened by karmic/hereditary factors—
which are the first to stash—and the first to suffer—
from my abusive lifestyle,
the first to warp and manifest symptoms,
within either themselves or a child or children;
even in "perfect" health, my target organs remain—
waiting . . .

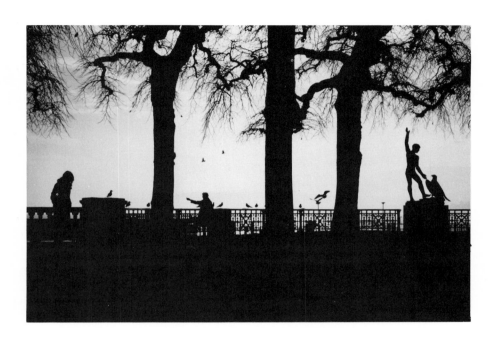

38

Condensed bioenergy seeks liberation and freedom—
my bodymind seeks balance and harmony,
seeks release from dis-ease and its symptoms;
a symptom—while indicating a crisis within—
is also proof positive that my bodymind is healing,
and purging, and cleansing itself of karma,
is unwarping, unkinking my organ/meridian system—
all symptom syndromes are **healing crises**.

A symptom may manifest physically as pain,
mentally, as emotional distress—
yet each begins in my karmic/intuitive sheath,
each is purged through my organ/meridian system,
each first burns karma stashed in its home organs,
but affects me totally as the crisis continues.

It is neither dis-ease nor symptoms that kill me—
only my failure to properly respond to a healing crisis.

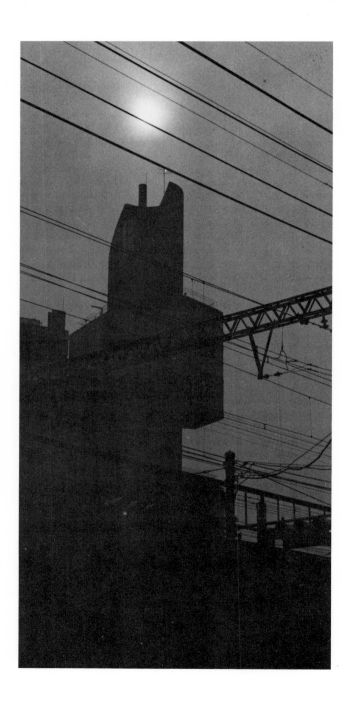

39

That I am becoming karmically charged—
paving the way for symptomatic purging and cleansing—
is apparent long before a symptom manifests overtly:
> *markings of my irises;*
> *color and hue of my complexion and aura;*
> *my hungers and cravings;*
> *the words I speak, my tone of voice;*
> *lines and wrinkles of distress on my extremities;*
> *my choice of activities and entertainment;*
> *the state of my many pulses;*
> *tenderness of various acupoints;*
> *sores or blemishes on specific parts of my skin;*
> *the smells and sounds I emit;*
> *my responses to various stimulii;*
> *pain around or within afflicted organs . . .*

There are many indicators of my state of health,
mirrors reflecting the path my well-being is likely to take;
the symptom I finally manifest is the last—
the most obvious and gross—
statement that my ways are unwise.

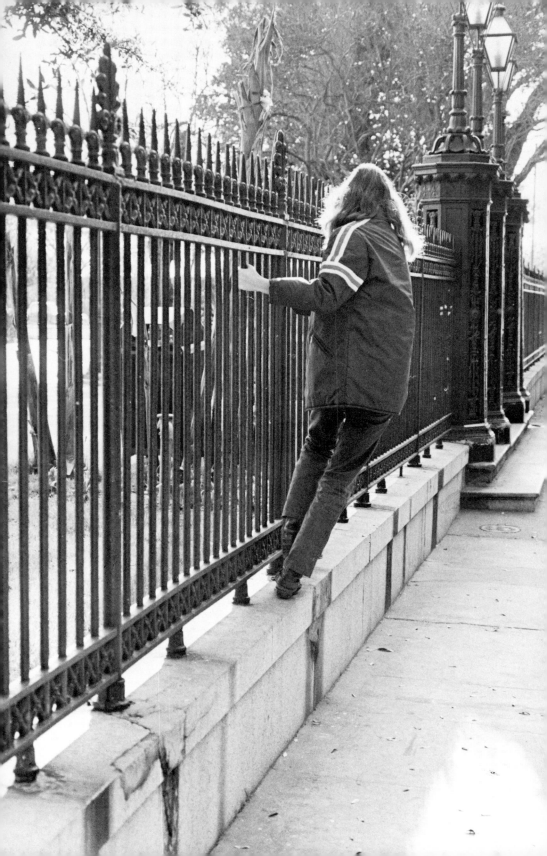

40

Freedom and subtlety, the superior—
condensed and rigid, the inferior;
mind is more subtle and free than the body—
thus, it dominates and reigns supreme.

As my mind weakens—or strengthens—
so my body must follow;
there is no imaginary illness or symptom:
I am ill if I think I am ill.

And that which prevents utter chaos within
is the hope and belief I can truly survive,
even in my darkest of moments.

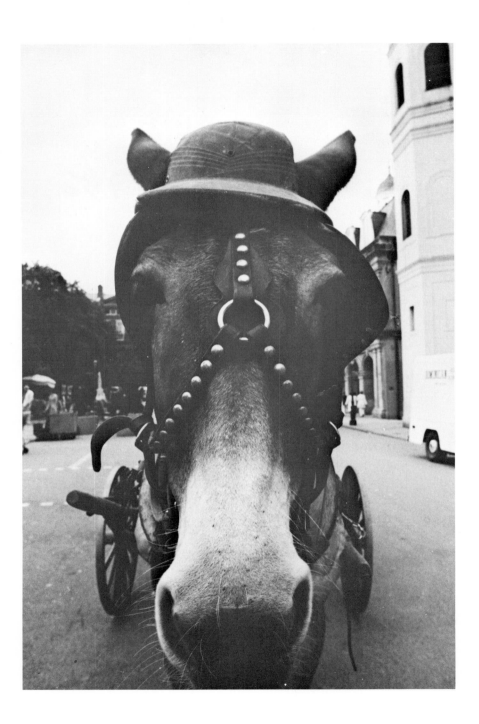

41

Ego sprouts from the karmic "seed"
I carry back into this incarnation;
ego—the most basic of my fear responses—
seeks shelter and protection
before the general welfare of my bodymind;
thus, I tend to choose repression and karma
by avoiding responsibility for my foolishness,
for my ignorance, for my abuse—
if ego, alone, dominates my decisions,
I can expect dis-ease instead of "loss of face,"
and symptoms instead of the objective self-assessment
that must precede—and continually accompany—
the returning to—and the maintenance of—
my state of good health.

My karmic burden grows and multiplies
as pieces of straw placed upon a camel's back—
thus, it is said that ego is the root of suffering,
ego is the source of dis-ease,
ego is both parent and child of karma, and rebirth,
and rebirth . . .

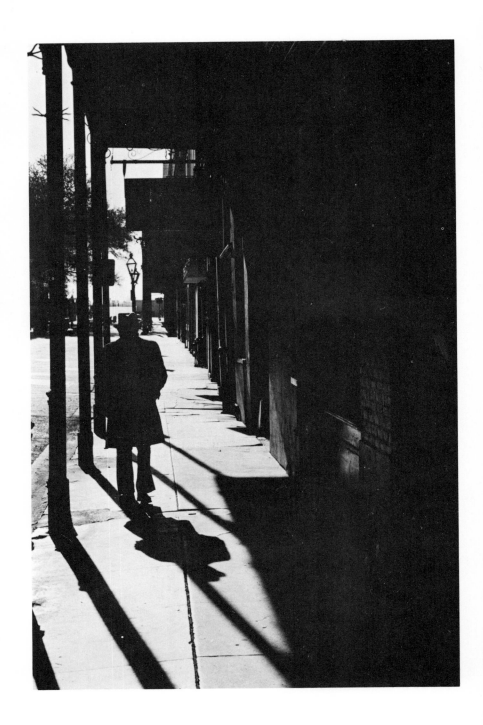

42

Health is a relative state of being, not absolute—
I can move *toward* or *away from* perfectly balanced bioflow,
but in the physical realm I am never perfectly healthy,
never totally balanced, never fully at ease.

I began this incarnation with a karmic "debt"—
as I age, moving from the yang of youth toward yin,
it is natural for my organs to gradually warp;
as my ego inflates and becomes offended or pampered,
I lure myself, tempt myself, fantasize and lead myself
into activities unhealthy, unwise . . .

While I may retard *aging* by a healthy lifestyle—
or accelerate the erosion by one foolish and profane—
this cycle, this incarnation, must complete itself;
there is no physical or mental immortality—
no total freedom from suffering and dis-ease.

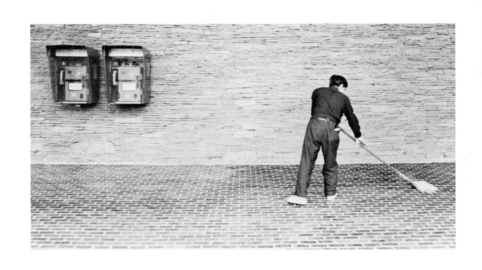

43

I, alone, created my dis-ease—
I, alone, am responsible for my healing;
*I am self-healing and **only** I can heal myself.*

Just as my actions may constantly generate karma,
so my reactions may constantly purge it:
Physical symptoms and mental distress—these are healing;
dreaming is healing, and crying, as well—
scratching unconsciously at "itchy" acupoints,
being injured, exhaling, excreting,
apologizing . . . laughing . . .

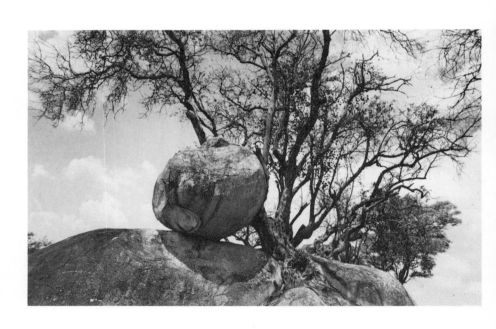

44

Healing is always by degrees, never by absolutes:
Healing, evolution, liberation—one, single process;
the only way it can be retarded, even temporarily reversed,
is by my ignorant or deliberate abuse,
by my refusal to flow with changing conditions.

If I wish to release a handful of sand,
all I need do is open my hand—
the sand takes care of itself;
and to heal myself, all I need to do is **stop the abuse.**

If I wish to accelerate the healing process
I can take a more aggressive step:
I can apply a **therapy**, a *counter*-abuse;
if abuse triggers a symptom to manifest itself,
the right counter-abuse—the right therapy—
may stimulate my bodymind to heal itself;
but while a counter-abuse may be therapeutic,
no therapy is complete until I *stop the abuse.*

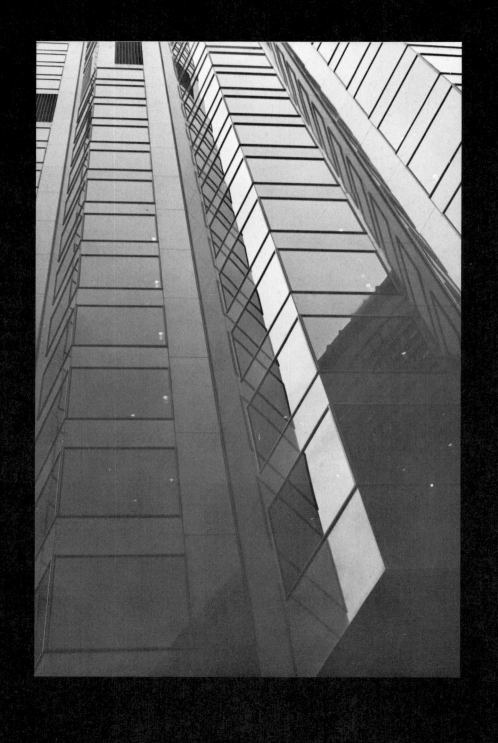

45

The goal of any therapy, any counter-abuse,
is to manipulate and alter the flow of free bioenergy
away from imbalance, *toward* balance and harmony.

Just as there are certain basic abuses
from which all abuses must extend,
so, too, there are **five, basic methods**
for therapeutically changing bioflow:
> *physically*—*massage, breath control, exercise* . . .
> *mechanically*—*acupuncture, surgery* . . ..
> *biologically*—*antibodies, vaccines* . . .
> *chemically*—*drugs, foods, herbs and teas* . . .
> *psychically*—*meditation, apology, hypnosis, prayer* . . .

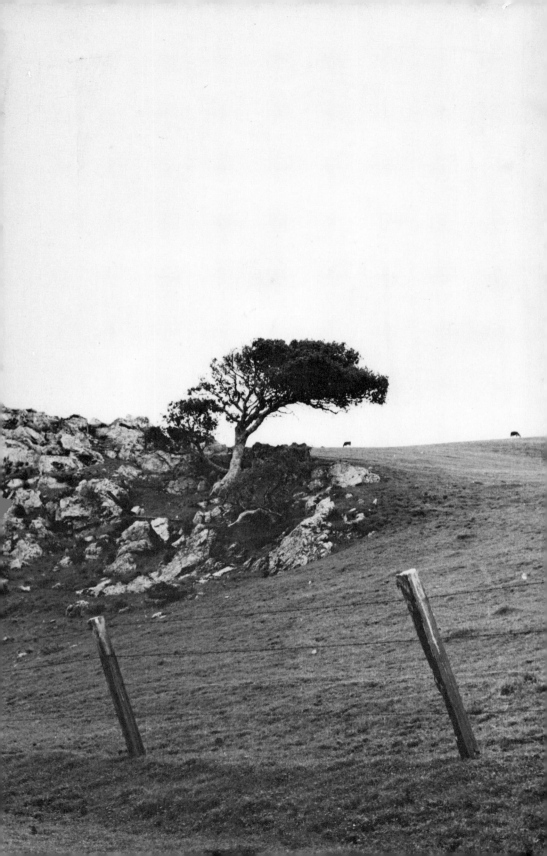

46

The single dis-ease—imbalanced bioflow—
has **four "sub-diseases"**—*divisions of illness*—
within one of which each symptom must fall:
>   ***excess yang;***
>   ***excess yin;***
>   ***deficient yang;***
>   ***deficient yin.***

The proper therapy adds to the deficiency—
or subtracts from the excess—
regardless of the method or means.

A sound, a weed, a cup of mud . . .
each thing has its quality and character,
its bioenergetic "vibrational tone,"
more yang or more yin than my own—
thus, there are many possible antidotes
for my excess or deficiency of yang or yin influence.

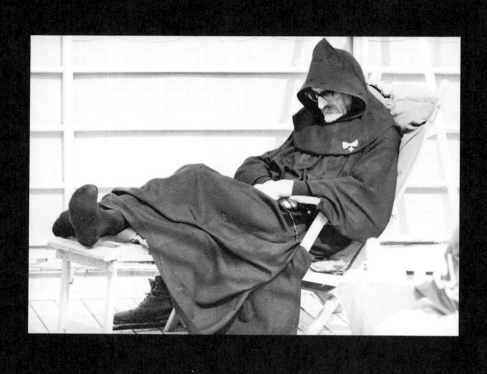

47

Each physical symptom has its mental distress,
just as all mental symptoms can finally be traced
to at least one physical organ;
thus, there is no panacea—
the right therapy for any symptom syndrome
is that which works best.

The more subtle and gentle the therapy,
the less obvious and immediate its results—
yet the more subtle and gentle the therapy,
the more pervasive its benefits
and the more totally it moves into my karmic/intuitive sheath.

But each therapy finally affects my entire bodymind,
however slowly or quickly, however long-lasting its results.

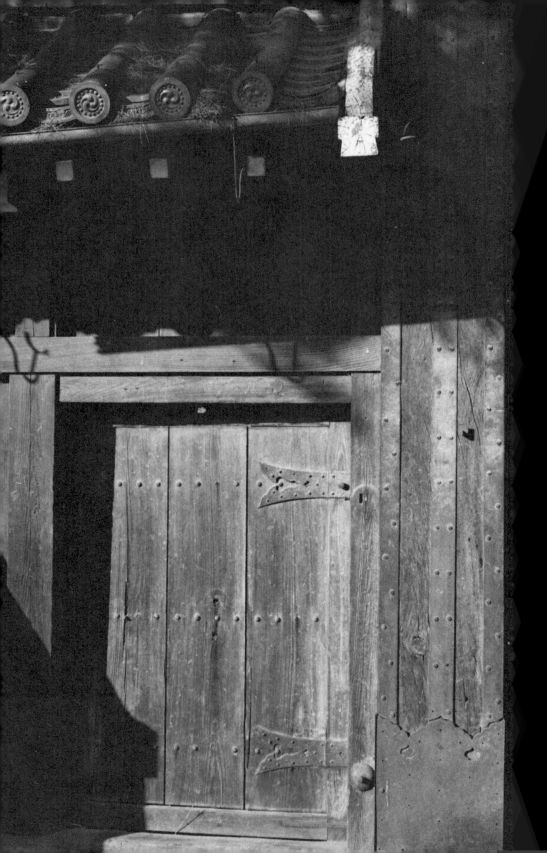

48

Each symptom syndrome has many phenomena—
pain, fever, germs, emotionality, distress . . .

Therapeutically changing even one aspect
of my symptom syndrome's many faces
may allow my bodymind to hasten its chore
of self-healing and evolution;
a house has many doors and windows—
each may provide access to the entire dwelling,
regardless of what room is first entered,
and by whichever opening entrance is first gained.

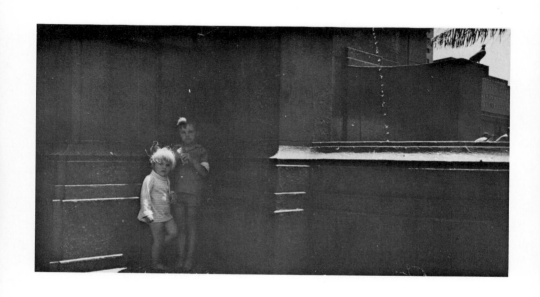

49

That which is an abuse to my bodymind
may be a counter-abuse to my brother's;
every thing, every activity, within and around me
has an abusive or counter-abusive quality,
regardless how subtle or harsh—
and, since the nature of living is ceaseless change,
that which heals me today may harm me tomorrow,
while that which is not healing and liberating
must be, by default, sickening and karmic—
there is no standing still—there is no status quo.

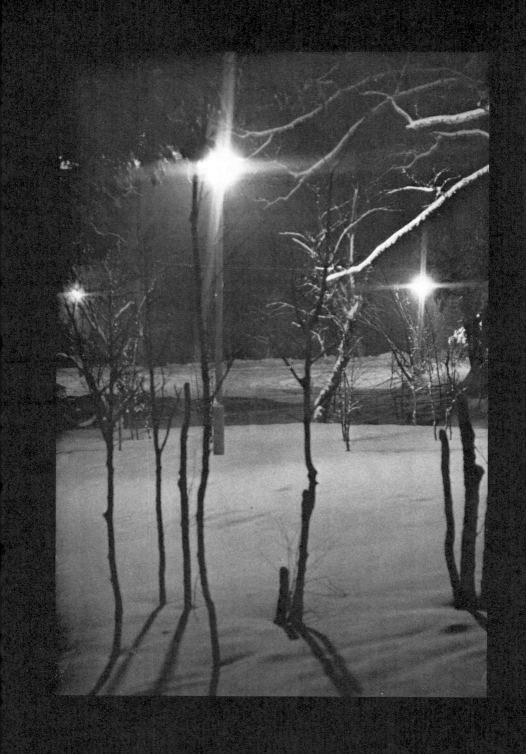

50

Good therapy includes **three, vital aspects:**
> *It relieves suffering;*
> *it shows where imbalance lies;*
> *it reveals the abuses that led to dis-ease.*

Therapy without diagnosis: Can this be called therapy?

Any therapy, counter-abuse or healing technique
is but a provisional measure, its results temporary;
but as my abuses are dropped or corrected,
my bioflow becomes balanced and my symptoms depart—
water cannot overflow from a half-filled vessel,
fire cannot burn without fuel . . .

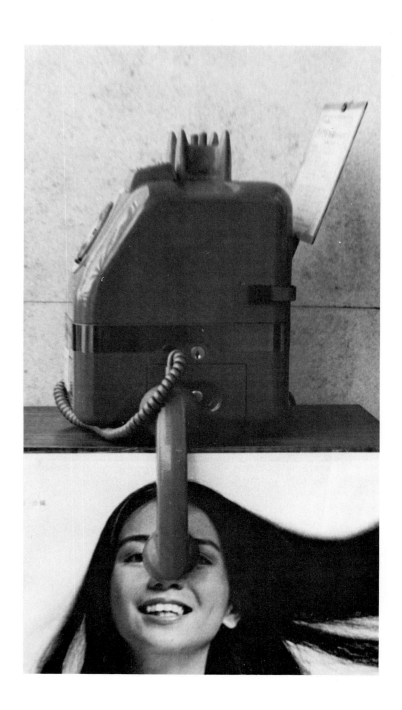

51

Even the best—the most appropriate—
therapy for any symptom,
falls as a seed on a bed of gravel
unless I, the sufferer, wish my suffering ended—
*to get well, I must first **want** to get well.*

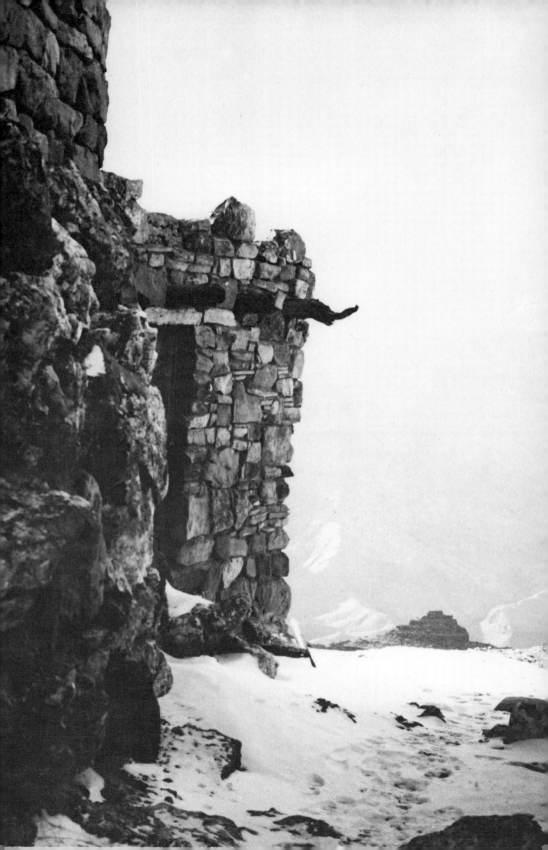

52

As my aura and organs become karmically "charged,"
only a minor abuse may trigger an **acute symptom**—
one with a "brushfire" quality—
harsh, painful, intense, brief . . .

My dis-ease progresses, my consciousness "clouds"—
I *appear* to heal, yet forget the state of vibrant well-being
that characterized my days of good health;
in my aging I become *chronically* ill,
suffering periodic outbursts of symptoms
as my organ/meridian system struggles to cope;
step by step, my dis-ease becomes *degenerative,*
then *debilitating,*
until, finally, my bodymind dies—
that is the path of dis-ease.

Dis-ease—and its symptoms—heal in reverse:
I often get **"worse"**—
relive and complete the traumas I've stashed—
especially the most painful—the acute—phase of dis-ease—
before I am healed;
if I stray from the mountain's path by five steps,
it takes five steps to return to the path—
if I stray by ten steps, then ten steps to return . . .

That is the path of healing.

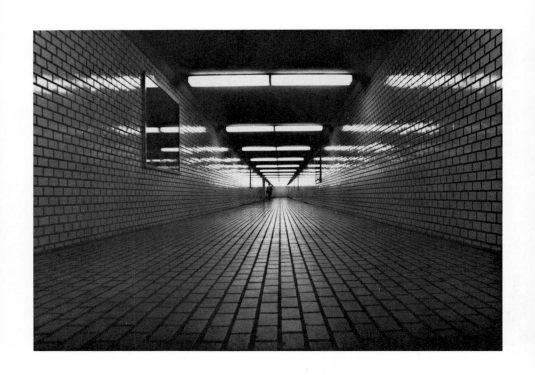

53

My organs warp and change—they do not "wear out";
thus, unless my bodymind is already too weakened
to tolerate the traumas of a healing crisis,
any symptom I manifest can, as well, be reversed—
there are no incurable symptoms and illnesses.

Dis-ease is most easily reversed and healed
in its earliest—its "pre-acute"—phase;
it is always more healthy for me to control,
to counter—to voluntarily stop—my abuses
while still in the state of relatively good health,
than be forced into change upon being terrorized
by a severe symptom syndrome manifesting itself.

The weaker, more dis-eased I am,
the more traumatic the healing process must be;
thus, it takes an intense commitment to reverse my dis-ease—
with its accompanying turbulence—
at a time when my determination and strength
are at their lowest ebb . . .

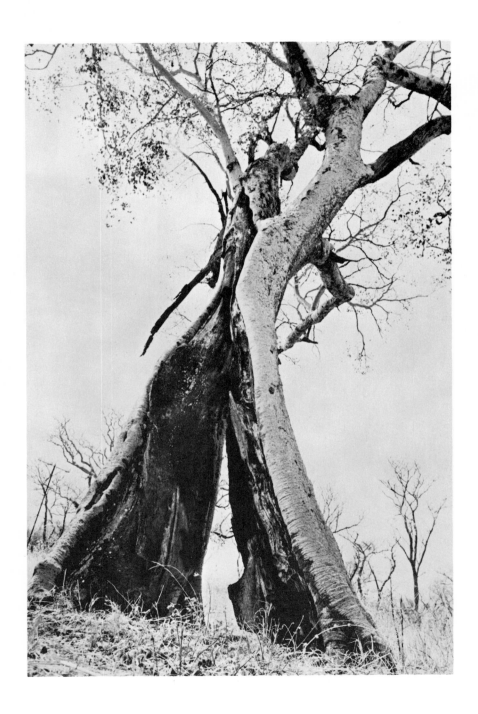

54

The more dis-eased and imbalanced my state of health
the faster I initially respond to therapy;
the more distressed my bodymind becomes,
the more anxiously it seeks to restore itself to balance;
the further from harmony my bioflow is "stretched,"
the less is required to begin the process of healing;
thus, when I am ill, even the gentlest of therapies—
perhaps nothing more than a suggestion—
becomes enough to start reversing dis-ease.

But for the process to continue, once set into motion,
my abuses must be countered, then stopped,
my acupoints relaxed and my organs unwarped
as the burning of karma proceeds at its pace—
karma is the root of my illness;
my illness is finished when its karma is burned.

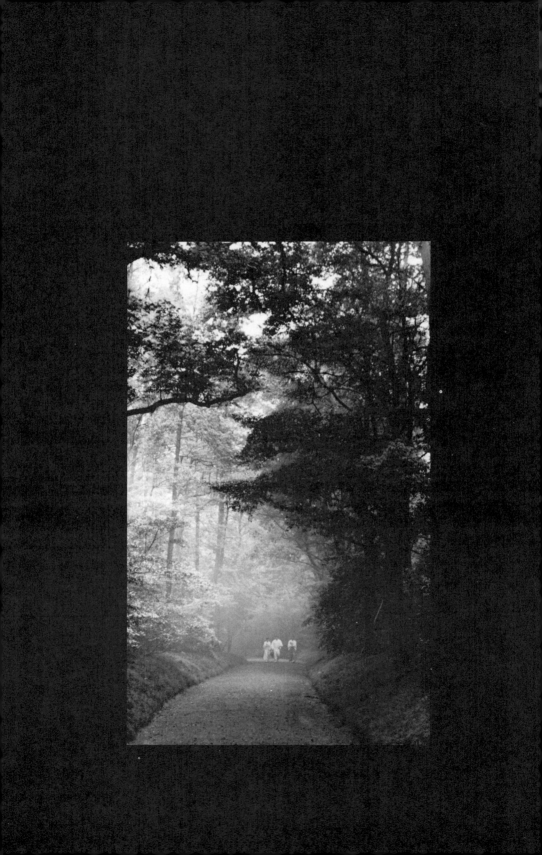

55

I am drawn toward **enlightenment**—
the unburdened state of understanding—and surrendering to—
the natural laws of the universe—
by the process of evolution;
though I may hinder my growth by refusing to flow,
I only generate karma and dis-ease in reaction.

Karma is the problem toward which I am pulled,
its solution is the way my karma is burned—
I cannot escape my karma,
but I may burn it in many ways;
the more unenlightened I choose to remain,
the more likely it is that my ego will choose "getting sick"
rather than the embarassment of being exposed as a fool;
and the more chronic my dis-ease becomes,
the fewer become my options for purging and cleansing;
the more dis-eased and imbalanced my bioflow network,
the more necessary becomes its purging through symptoms.

Yet dis-ease and its symptoms are stopgaps—not cures;
I condemn myself to repeated symptoms, repeated incarnations,
until the message of my imbalance becomes clear:
>   *My ego, my desires, my attachments,*
>   *cannot be protected without great emotional expense;*
>   *and their ultimate loss—*
>   *with or without my cooperation—*
>   *is assured.*

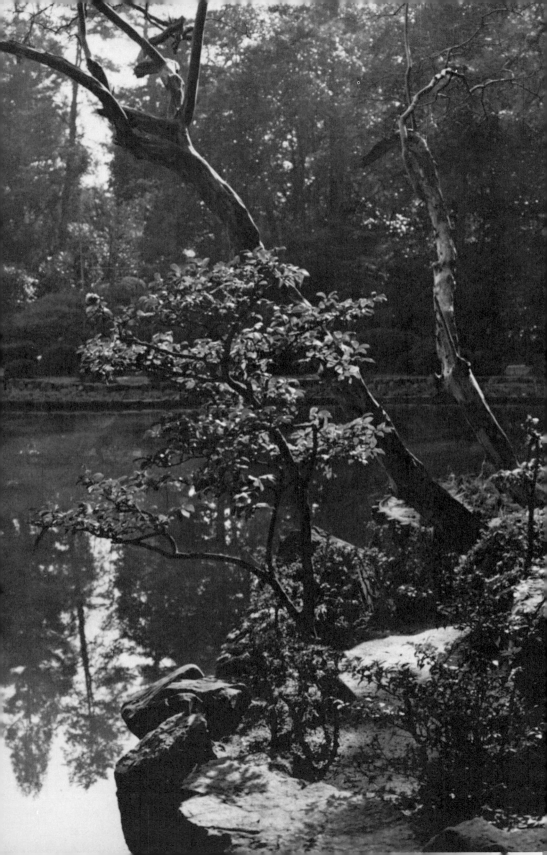

56

The more healthy I become,
the more quickly I respond to change;
the more my consciousness unclouds,
the greater becomes my sense of perspective—
healing—like suffering—is a holistic syndrome of reactions.

Thus, the more balanced my bioflow becomes,
the lighter grows my karmic burden
and the less abuse it takes to return me
to the painful state of chaos, the acute phase of dis-ease;
the more karmically cleansed I become,
the more quickly I burn any new karma
I generate through my unwise activities.

The closer I move toward balanced bioflow,
the more increasingly subtle—yet pervasive—
become the results of my therapies and prevention—
each karmic stash that I burn
removes yet another "cloud layer" from my consciousness;
step by step I become enlightened,
become my own doctor, become my own patient,
become aware of each of my actions,
each of my thoughts, each bite of food . . .

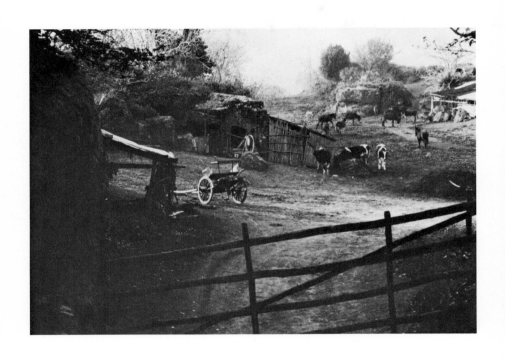

57

Free will—a vital ingredient of abuse and karma—
is essential for generating dis-ease and imbalance;
likewise, free will is crucial for healing:
Through free will I may recognize the desirability
of changing actions and attitudes that led to dis-ease;
and only through my power of choice
can I make the commitment—and apply the techniques—
to reverse my imbalance and return toward good health.

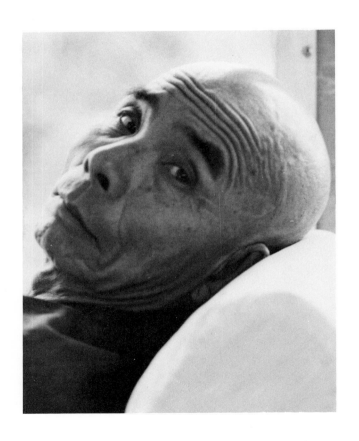

58

Conscious evolution is aided and quickened
by strengthening trust in my sense of intuition—
I can never have enough factual knowledge
to make a completely rational decision;
but the natural laws governing each situation
reveal themselves clearly, intuitively—
if I allow that to happen.

But freely or haltingly, I must become enlightened,
though it may take a million lifetimes—
my stubborness and refusal to unburden myself
is of no consequence within the bounds of the universe,
for nothing is ever lost or misplaced . . .

Yet I can instantly drop the clouds from my consciousness—
I am already enlightened, my soul is free—
I only cling to the attachment and illusion I am burdened—
but fear of loss, fear of the unknown, fear of death,
keeps my soul bound to this realm,
keeps me chained to this condensed, yin plane of existence,
this **purgatory**—
this place for purging and burning my karma.

健

康

之

道

PART III

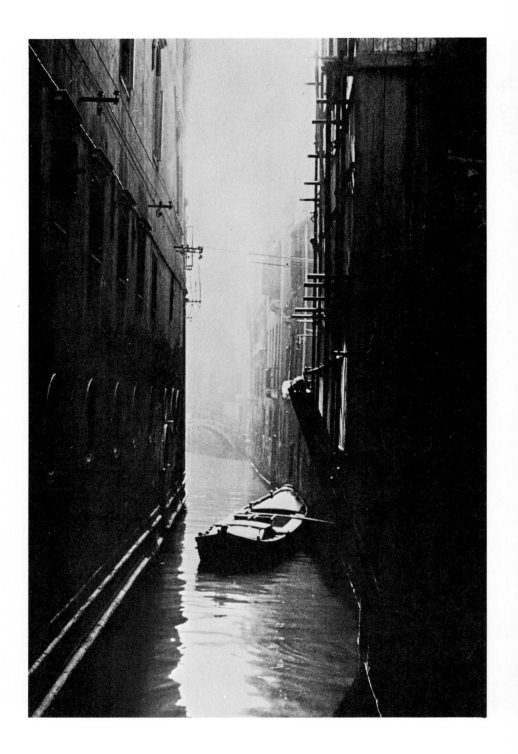

59

Strengthen the hara,
be wary of karma;
surrender the ego
while following dharma.

This is the way of healing,
the path to health, enlightenment and freedom
as prescribed by traditional healers of the East . . .

. . . Strengthen the *hara*—

hara: Most powerful spot of my bodymind,
          yet the most vulnerable—
          two inches below my navel,
          second lowest of my *chakras,*
          wellspring of my animal vitality,
          root of this physical incarnation;

hara: Focus of the **"superior therapies"**—
          breath control and meditation—
          when my *hara* is strong and supple,
          the rest of my bodymind must follow;
          but when my *hara* is rigid or weak,
          dis-ease cannot be reversed . . .

. . . be wary of karma—

As two dissimilar straight lines must eventually cross,
so my bodymind, moving from yang to yin,
must finally converge with my karmic accumulation—
the exhausting burden of my ignorance and abuses—
striking the death-knell of this incarnation.

Hara—only the center of this bodymind,
only the focus of this incarnation—
is inferior to my karma;
even strong and supple,
my hara *must surrender to the force of my karma.*

As a man without a country
sails from foreign shore to foreign shore,
so each bodymind I manifest
carries me across the stormy sea of physical life,
a lonely captain in search of his port;
until my karma is totally burned,
I manifest vessel after vessel—
pretty ones, ugly ones, healthy ones, dis-eased . . .

. . . surrender the ego—

Without ego, no karma—
without ego, no reincarnation,
no bodymind, no *hara*, no dis-ease nor decay.

Surrender:
>*The moment of climax in sexual orgasm . . .*
>*releasing myself into sleep . . .*
>*deep meditation . . .*
>*begging . . .*

Surrender, to be complete, is both constant and voluntary;
but could I tolerate the ecstasy of endless orgasm?
Or want to sleep for the rest of my life?
Or meditate—even beg?
Or in any other way lose all thought of self?

Yet each act of surrender brings me a glimpse
of the way to concluding my whole karmic cycle:
And no surrender, no conclusion—
the choice is always mine . . .

. . . while following *dharma*—

No voids, no emptiness—
as the thunderhead dissolves, clear sky takes its place;
as my ego crumbles, my soul "expands"—
yet to exist socially without ego is . . . nearly impossible.

But every front must have its backside,
and every action, its reaction;
thus, in my weakness lies my strength—
in my karma lies my *dharma*—
my true path to enlightenment,
my reason and purpose for this incarnation,
the knotted, jumbled thread, that—
with patience and commitment—
I may unravel to terminate my karmic cycle.

As surely as I become dis-eased through karmic activities,
so I cleanse my organ/meridian system
through *counter*-karmic tasks—
dharmic chores that carry the seed of enlightenment,
the work—simple and menial or complex and "important"—
that I must do to fulfill my own destiny;
as a wanderer stumbling lost in a cave,
revels upon finding, again, his homeward-bound path,
so, in returning to *dharma*—my own, special way—
I sense pleasure, correctness—my life feels complete.

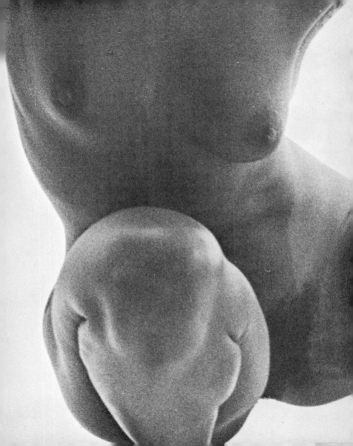

60

I am a descendent of Tao's division—
yang and yin are my ancestors;
I incarnate from lifetime to lifetime,
doomed to wander the ages
'til I choose to leap from this treadmill
by surrendering resistance to the nature of Tao.

The way—the single way—to spring from this karmic carousel
is to finally surrender the yin-most part of my being—
attachment to emotions, dis-ease, ego, karma—
to the yang-most—*my soul—*
as I retrace the path of Tao's division.

All therapy eventually leads to "spiritual surrender";
no therapy is complete without it.

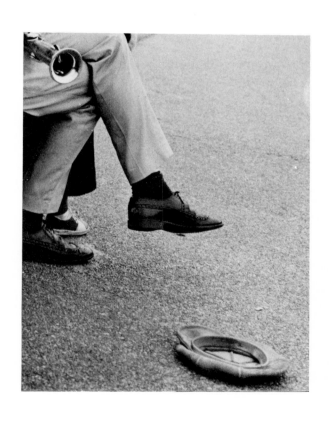

61

The belief that I hold in my own capabilities
must falter at some point in the process of aging;
belief in my self, alone, nourishes ego,
adds karmic weight to my burden.

So easy, so easy—
nothing required to surrender the ego—I could do it now!
Yet spiritual surrender is my supreme act of strength . . .

Surrender is eased by releasing my self
to a devotional "object" representing the superior—
a word, the wind, an icon or parent . . .

In the quest to identify my devotional object
I stumble across my **guru**—
my teacher, my source of direction,
my spiritual Master—
my vital-most step on the path to enlightenment.

I returned to the physical with my guru—
He is with me now, as always;
ten minutes, ten years, ten incarnations from now—
the timing is irrelevant—
I must allow my guru to reveal Himself,
it cannot fail to happen.

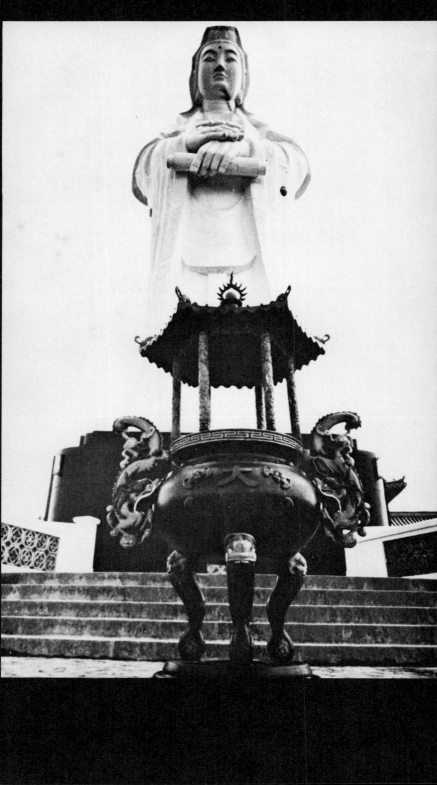

62

Just as I can accelerate healing with therapy,
accelerate karmic purging through *dharmic* chores,
accelerate evolution through spiritual surrender,
so, too, I can hasten my guru's revelation:
All I need do is recognize—and admit to myself—
that I no longer desire, nor feel I am able,
to cope with my burdens or deal with my loneliness . . .

These are the words to summon my guru:
      Please help me—I give up.

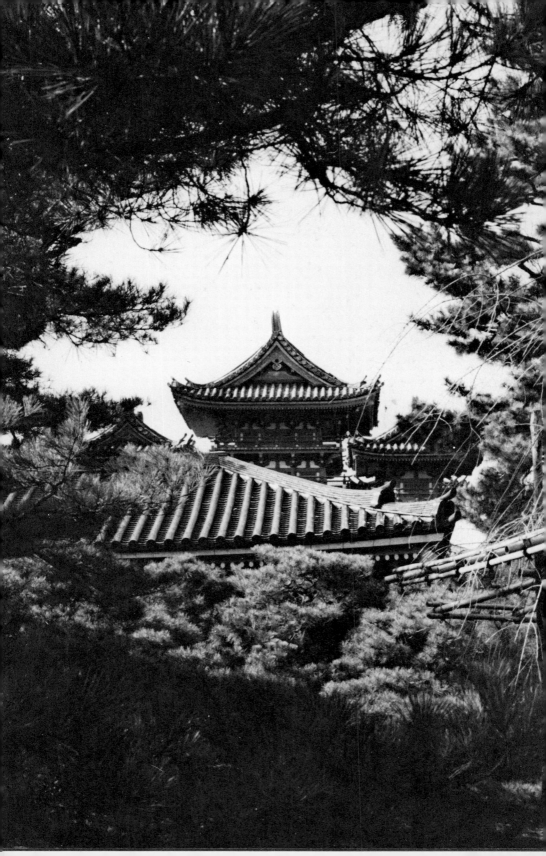

63

I may never glimpse my guru in the physical realm—
He may be long-since dead, it makes no difference:
Our rapport is psychic, our connection spans time and space;
the more completely I surrender to my Master,
the more my intuition is His voice, the less it is my own.

Spiritual surrender—an attitude, not an action—
eases the agony of aloneness,
quiets my terror when contemplating death;
the more completely I surrender my earthly priorities
to those of my guru, my teacher, my Master,
the more I am freed of my quest for immortality—
a state that is mine without striving for or earning—
and the more I am freed of my yearning for health.

Upon recognizing deep in my consciousness
the absolute truth of my need to surrender,
then, upon accepting this ultimate challenge,
I set into motion a subtle—but powerful—chain of phenomena:
My organ/meridian system begins self-correcting,
the state of my health soon starts to improve,
the tensions and stresses of life's many problems
are gently relieved as my balance returns—
I surrender to my guru—not for His sake—but for my own.

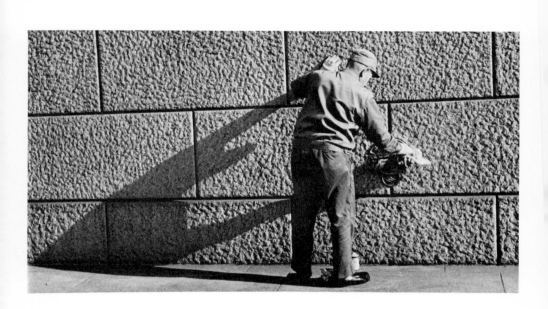

64

As my consciousness unclouds, as my burden is shed,
I become as one finger of my guru's countless hands,
performing His chores of selfless service as my own *dharma*,
becoming one of His countless voices echoing a single word:
    Love.

There is only love—nothing else:
Ego is selfless love warped by fear—fear of death;
karmic activities—love warped by expectations,
by disappointments, by unfulfilled yearnings;
there is no hatred, only love warped by ego—
there is no evil, only foolish ignorance of love.

Love—ceaseless, selfless, all-surrounding—
has many branches, many leaves:
My love for parents, family, children—
the hunger luring me to my sexual mate—
the devotion I feel for my guru and Master,
the respect that I hold for the life-forms around me—
yet the pleasure of success, the ecstasy of orgasm,
the surrender to devoted duty . . .
at the roots of each feeling is the tingle of unwarped bioflow—
at the roots of each feeling is love.

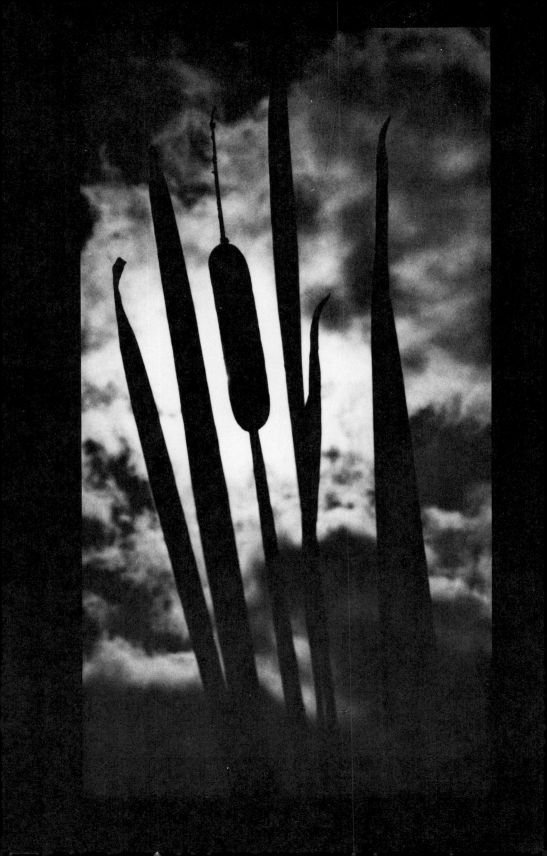

65

My *dharmic* path of least resistance
is the one that offers me the most pleasure,
for I can never totally enjoy a karmic activity—
and to the extent I can find guiltless pleasure
in even an activity I know is unwise,
to that same extent its karma is gentled;
thus, in choosing the ways of my life,
if my first thought is pleasure
I am bound to be lured toward my natural path.

The more completely I surrender my ego,
the more intuitively, the more lovingly,
the more pleasingly correct
are the choices I make in finding my way.

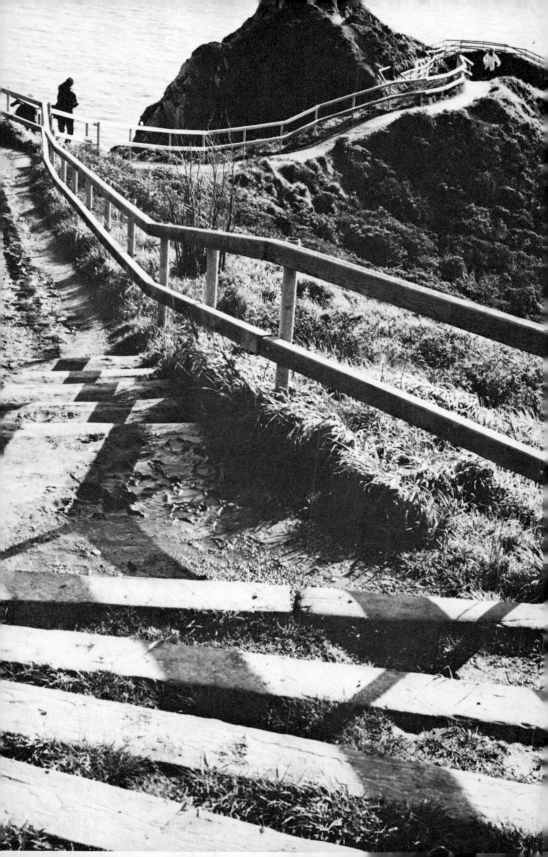

66

As I move toward enlightenment
I evolve to the "superior person" I am in my soul,
existing my full century—even longer, with care—
in pleasure and harmony within my surroundings;
deftly I move along my path,
surrendering to my microcosmic existence in time,
radiating love selflessly, ceaselessly—
touching some situations, avoiding others—
sensing my natural way as a brook finds the ocean,
bubbling, bubbling with laughter!

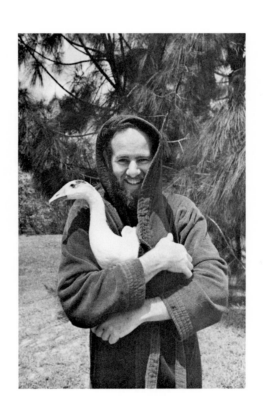

AFTERWORD

In writing THE TAO OF HEALTH—an amalgam of traditional Eastern healing and spiritual philosophies as I understand them—it has been my intention to explain the so-called "energy theory of dis-ease" in a manageable, if somewhat classical, format. The human bodymind is an intricate and complex mechanism; yet it truly does follow the prescripts described by the ancients of the East. A basic knowledge and understanding of these axioms seems essential for one's spiritual and psychophysical well-being—which are, of course, synonymous.

Michael Blate

MORE ABOUT THE PHOTOGRAPHS

Without exception, photographs in the preceding pages were shot with cameras and lenses from Nippon Kogaku K.K. (Nikon):

chapter and subject	lens	film
1 sunrise, Indian Ocean	24mm, f2.8	Plus-X
2 snail	55mm, f3.5	Tri-X
3 sunflower seeds	55mm	Tri-X
4 baobab tree, Tanzania	24mm	Plus-X
5 wood	55mm	Plus-X
6 rocks, Tanzania	105mm, f2.5	Plus-X
7 leaves	55mm	EktaChrome
8 New Mexico	55mm	Plus-X
9 girl, Labrador puppy	105mm	Tri-X
10 eggs	55mm	Tri-X
11 onion	55mm	Tri-X
12 Youth Fair, Dade County, Florida	24mm	KodaChrome
13 Singapore	105mm	Plus-X
14 Kyoto, Japan	55mm	Fuji
15 New Orleans	105mm	Tri-X
16 tai chi chu'an instructor, Hong Kong	55mm	Plus-X
17 Israel	24mm	Plus-X
18 Arizona	24mm	Plus-X
19 Nikko, Japan	55mm	Fuji
20 San Francisco	105mm	FujiChrome

51	phone booth, Tokyo	55mm	Fuji
52	Grand Canyon, Arizona	105mm	Plus-X
53	subway, Osaka, Japan	55mm	Fuji
54	Rhodesia	24mm	Plus-x
55	Tokyo	55mm	Fuji
56	Kyoto	55mm	Fuji
57	near Rome	50mm	AgfaChrome
58	Buddhist monk on train, near Taipei, Taiwan	105mm	Plus-X
59	Venice, Italy	50mm	Plus-X
60	torso	55mm	Tri-X
61	New Orleans	55mm	Tri-X
62	Taipei	24mm	Tri-X
63	Kyoto	55mm	Fuji
64	Tokyo	55mm	Fuji
65	cattails	55mm	Tri-X
66	Marin County, California	24mm	Tri-X
Afterword—author wearing goose and bathrobe (by Gail Watson)		24mm	Tri-X
Front cover—Israel		50mm	KodaChrome
Rear cover—Israel		50mm	KodaChrome

*For further information about natural health
and traditional Oriental healing techniques,
please contact:*

**THE G-JO INSTITUTE
POST OFFICE BOX 8060,
HOLLYWOOD, FLORIDA 33024**